Finding Joy

with an Invisible Chronic Illness

Proven Strategies for Discovering Happiness, Meaning, and Fulfillment

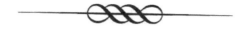

Christopher Martin

Library of Congress Control Number: 2021920945

Published in 2021 by Martin Family Bookstore

Martin Family Bookstore
Sauquoit, NY 13456
www.invisibleillnessbooks.com

Consider using the workbook by Oak Tree Reading on Amazon to enhance your reading experience. This could be useful for solo readers or support groups.

Printed in the United States of America

Hardcover ISBN: 9780990826941
Paperback ISBN: 9780990826958
eBook ISBN: 9780990826965
Audiobook ISBN: 9780990826989

Please note: This book is for informational purposes only and it is not a rendering of, or a substitute for, professional advice. Specific psychological, lifestyle, behavioral, medical, or nutritional needs require the services of a qualified healthcare professional. Furthermore, the case example at the start of chapter 4 is fictitious although it offers an accurate representation of someone who has experienced grief and loss. Additionally, I make no guarantee that the website links will stay functional over time, as many websites get changed, deleted, or moved. Further, as the author I make no guarantee, express or implied, regarding the recommendations discussed. Nor do I assume any liability regarding the consequences resulting from the use of the content in this book.

Finding Joy with an Invisible Chronic Illness is dedicated to all those who suffer from chronic illnesses, often misunderstood and in silence, many of whom feel depleted of hope, energy, and life.

Finding Joy with an Invisible Chronic Illness is also dedicated to those who have lost loved ones or suffered from chronic illness as a result of the coronavirus pandemic of 2020. Although the pandemic provided me the rare gift of time to write this book, my heart aches for the tremendous loss of life and suffering.

Praise for *Finding Joy*

"Chronic illness has the potential of allowing the individual to grow personally from the experience or become a victim and debilitated emotionally, physically, and spiritually. *Finding Joy* provides a comprehensive, evidence-based roadmap for not only coping with chronic illness, but personally optimizing self-growth and resiliency from the experience." —**Joanne Joseph, PhD**, professor of psychology and interim dean of the College of Health Sciences, SUNY Polytechnic Institute, and author of *The Resilient Child: Preparing Today's Youth for Tomorrow's World*

"*Finding Joy* is absolutely phenomenal. Chris Martin's heartfelt approach offers numerous meaningful strategies to thrive when faced with the many unseen and unrecognized issues of living with an invisible chronic illness." —**Heather Lewis-Hoover, MS, CAS**, school counselor

"This book offers great value for anyone with chronic illness as it contains clear, practical, and actionable insights and steps that can be naturally implemented into daily life. An engaging, easy, and helpful read. Highly recommended." —**Alla Bogdanova, MSc, MIM**, co-founder and past president of the International Empty Nose Syndrome Association

"*Finding Joy* is a vital guide on how to best manage and navigate life with a chronic illness." —**James Nestor**, *New York Times* bestselling author of *Breath: The New Science of a Lost Art*

"Chronic illness can leave you depleted of energy, withdrawn, full of self-blame, and wallowing in self-pity. You won't feel this way after reading this book! An easy-to-read, understand, and very useful resource, *Finding Joy* will not only lift your spirits, but it will also show you how to navigate the complex social and emotional journey of living with a chronic ailment." —**Kai Zhao, PhD**, associate professor, Department of Otolaryngology – Head & Neck Surgery, Ohio State University

"There are times in our lives when practical guidance is not only needed, but is provided in a way that lifts the greater good. From the unique vantage point of a patient and school psychologist, Chris offers a complete resource for those suffering from invisible chronic illnesses.

Encouraging a holistic approach to chronic illness, he thoroughly explores and critiques the positive psychology literature to offer numerous communicating, thinking, feeling, and behavioral approaches.

Additionally, Chris offers a chapter specifically for those who have a loved one with a chronic illness so they, too, can help their chronically ill loved ones on their journey.

Having known Chris for decades, I am beyond fortunate to have been privy to such a work that serves others by providing a timely message, a powerhouse of practical strategies, and invaluable guidance." —**Mark Montgomery, PhD**, chief diversity officer, SUNY Polytechnic Institute, and founder and chair of Joseph's Experience, Inc., an organization that assists children impacted by cancer and/or leukemia

"While there is plenty of information here about acceptance, self-compassion, reappraisal, encouraging self-talk, social support, and positive psychology concepts and stress management techniques, the heart of this discussion lies in putting these ethereal concepts and ideals into daily life and interactions with others.

Anyone with chronic illness needs this blueprint of new pathways to joy. It's a survey recommended not just for the chronically ill patient, but also for the family and friends supporting their efforts." —**Diane Donavan**, senior reviewer, Midwest Book Review

"Life-changing. This book was beneficial to me because I suffer from chronic pain daily. I'm still in agony, but this book has greatly aided me." —**Tim Antonie on Amazon.com**

"This book was a great encouragement to me that in spite of my pain and suffering, I can still live an abundant life." —**Bob on Amazon.com**

"*Finding Joy* covers all aspects of what life is like living with a chronic illness, what to expect, how to deal with pitfalls, how to accept your illness, and how (utilizing psychology-based practices) to embrace and maximize the quality of your life in your 'new normal.'" —Ben H. on Amazon.com

"I've had an illness since age 14 and I still suffer from illness now. The author has some great tips and tricks for dealing with illness, in general, and [for] the mental health of someone with a chronic illness. A must read for anyone with an invisible chronic illness." —Carey's Reviews on Goodreads.com

"I have had various invisible chronic illnesses for nearly forty years, [but] I was still able to find suggestions that will help me. So many of the things I have gone through are reflected in this book. I highly recommend this comprehensive book." —Sue on Amazon.ca

"If you share his Christian faith, trust in God. Your illness is not your fault! There are many books, written by people of every faith, which promise that their deity can work miracles if you spend a few dollars, but this is not one of them. The roots of this book lie in the author's own suffering and how he tackled it. It is *jam-packed with advice* on how to get the treatment and support you need, both physical and emotional.

Never mind 'take up your bed and walk,' the miracle of JOY in my life lies within this book, and that is my new goal." —Sarah Stuart, Readers' Favorite reviewer

This is a book everyone should own as we are all likely to be or know someone we care about with chronic illness. This book provides opportunities for healing for absolutely every perspective. Covering spirituality, psychology, and biomechanics this book has it all. Though written from a Christian perspective the book is still very accessible and useful to other religious beliefs. I will be recommending this book to my clients." —T. Satterfield on Goodreads.com

"Christopher does a brilliant job of explaining the tools for managing the social, spiritual, mental, and physical aspects of chronic illness. I loved that the book contains straightforward tips for patients, their caregivers, and loved ones. Every chapter includes useful advice." — Edith Wairimu, Readers' Favorite reviewer

"Finding Joy with an Invisible Chronic Illness is a great find, one for all to read, the patient, the loved one, and family members. It is a simple and very practical approach to taking control by understanding how we think and what we have control over when it comes to our chronic condition and healthcare treatment." —**Melinda Sandor, Looking for the Light Blog**

"I really found the book to have great content, easy to read, helpful and interesting. I loved the section on grief, I thought the explanations of the different types of therapy were excellent, and the section on stress had very interesting information, not just a repeat of what we always hear. I also liked that he added the section on well-spouses and caregivers. I think the needs of those who take care of people with chronic illnesses are easily and often overlooked and this was a very important topic that he raised awareness about. Overall this book is a compilation of a lot of great info presented in a very effective manner.

One thing done really well: While many of the strategies presented in the book may be familiar to the reader, the author did a superb job of supplying additional information regarding these topics that is both interesting and not readily found in most self-help articles and books." —**Elizabeth Wells of Oak Tree Reading**

"This is about as close as anyone can get to a comprehensive list of options for dealing with chronic illnesses. It's very well organized and accessible. It's well written and easy to understand." —**Daniel B. Lyle on Amazon.com**

"As someone with chronic illness this book made me feel seen and understood, it was insightful and honest. The author covers many techniques that have successfully helped me manage my illness over the years, one amongst many others being pacing and how to practice it. He covers how we can use psychology, spirituality, supplements, stress management techniques, etc. to our benefit. There is a section on considerations for people with chronic illness in regard to exercise which I thought was great! This book takes a very holistic approach to living with chronic illness which is absolutely essential." —**Saira A. on NetGalley**

"This is the perfect book for people with chronic illness." —**Jay Rocken on Amazon.ca**

Table of Contents

Finding Joy

with an Invisible Chronic Illness

Proven Strategies for Discovering

Happiness, Meaning, and Fulfillment

Christopher Martin

Foreword

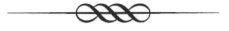

By Dr. Subinoy Das

A s a physician who treats a rare chronic illness, I have met patients from all over the world who suffer from both the devastating physical limitations of chronic disease, and also from the profound psychological, social, and interpersonal impacts. What has struck me is that despite the varied cultural influences that establish their worldview and foundational paradigms, my patients suffer a remarkably similar and expansive constellation of predicaments and ailments.

I have also noticed how poorly the medical profession and society at-large prepares people to deal with the tremendous breadth of suffering that chronic illness creates in all aspects of life.

Chris Martin recognizes this pervasive gap in our care for people with chronic illness. In this outstanding book, he details many of the different aspects of suffering that a chronic illness creates but, more importantly, provides a concise, well-researched guide on how to deal with this suffering and find joy and happiness in spite of it. He leans on both his experience as a chronic illness sufferer as well as a practicing school psychologist, father, and husband to provide concise, but thoroughly researched solutions.

In particular, his chapters on how to seek healthcare and efficiently make the best use of physician appointments dramatically provide a large return on investment from reading this book, especially for those who have been frustrated with the endless referrals, navigation, expense, and dissonance required to find high quality medical care.

Additionally, the chronically ill will benefit tremendously from sections on positive psychology and stress management. This book provides a practical guide to both confront the altered mindset that a chronic illness can create, as well as to engage in adaptive behaviors in dealing with chronic illness.

This book is also enormously useful for the insights that it provides to loved ones of those suffering from chronic illness. It is remarkably painful to watch a family member, dear friend, or loved one suffer in so many aspects of their life, and many feel unsure how they can help.

Chris provides a much-needed service in writing this exceptional book which offers its readers a powerful guidebook and weapon against the suffering associated with chronic illness. His comprehensive approach is what is needed. His readers, like me, will be much better off by learning from these insights gained from decades of experience in dealing with chronic disease.

Subinoy Das, MD, FACS, FARS, is CEO and director of the US Institute for Advanced Sinus Care & Research. A leading national surgeon, Dr. Das has received multiple America's Best Doctors awards, and he has been voted as one of the nation's top 5% of surgeons. His National Institutes of Health (NIH) funded research was awarded the 2013 Fowler Award (a top research award in otolaryngology) for his work on detecting the cause of sinus infections. Dr. Das suffers from chronic sinusitis following a baseball injury and suboptimal surgery.

Introduction

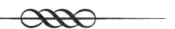

As if dealing with a debilitating chronic medical condition is not grueling enough. Your unremitting, tormenting chronic illness drains your time, energy, and ambition, impacting all aspects of your life. You find yourself in survival mode and inevitably confront a flood of negative thoughts and emotions ranging from shame and guilt for not doing more to feeling like you are letting others down to internalizing judgmental criticism from others. In so doing, the person you seem to fight the most emotional battles with is yourself.

Thanks to your illness, you also struggle in relating to others. Friends, family, co-workers – or even your healthcare professionals – question the severity of your condition and offer recommendations ranging from "Stay positive" to "But you look good" to "Try this 'cure' for your ailment." This well-intentioned, but misguided advice only compounds your misery, making you withdraw.

On top of that, accessing and maintaining high quality medical care for your condition poses its own sets of challenges. You may have more questions than answers about your illness. You may not be sure how to make the most of your brief appointment. You may not have a team of doctors working together on your behalf. Or your doctor may not be well-attuned to your specific needs.

It does not have to be this way.

You can take ownership of your physical and mental health, your relationships, and your life. You can stop negative thoughts and emotions in their tracks. Your relationships matter and, while you may not be able to control what others say to you, you can still enjoy satisfying relationships. You are not only worthy of respect from others, but from yourself as well. And you can obtain clarity on your medical condition and access quality medical care to manage it.

In short, you can take an intentional, holistic approach to managing chronic illness while not letting it overtake your life. By changing your thoughts and actions, by cultivating your relationships, and by taking the right steps toward understanding your condition and accessing quality medical care, you can improve your life. *Finding Joy* will show you how.

What Exactly is an Invisible Chronic Illness?

An invisible chronic illness is a debilitating physical ailment which:

1. Others do not readily observe;

2. Continues for a long period of time;

3. Impacts sufferers to varying degrees. It might be mildly debilitating with no or limited impact to work, relationships, or activities of daily living, while other illnesses wreak havoc on careers, hobbies, socialization, and daily life activities. For example, half of U.S. adults have a chronic medical condition, 96% of which are invisible, and about 10% of U.S. adults have a condition that impairs them in their daily life activities *to the extent* that it is considered an invisible disability;[1-2] this is the ideal reader for this book.

4. Debilitates on a continuous or constant basis. Further, the level of debilitation is unpredictable and variable.

5. Remains stable or progresses;

6. Includes fatigue, pain, brain fog, breathing difficulties, infections, irritable bowels, and/or neurological dysfunction. One may not always be acutely sick, but ongoing symptoms and struggles make them feel far from healthy.

Thousands of invisible illnesses exist. Examples include:

- Chronic fatigue syndrome (CFS)
- Celiac disease
- Sleep apnea
- Complex regional pain syndrome (CRPS)
- Cancer
- Heart disease
- Fibromyalgia
- Lupus
- Cystic Fibrosis
- Multiple sclerosis (MS)
- Ehlers-Danlos syndrome (EDS)
- Mental illness
- Post-traumatic stress disorder (PTSD)
- Traumatic brain injury (TBI)
- Arthritis
- Lyme disease
- Autoimmune disease
- Diabetes
- Hypothyroidism
- Epilepsy
- Asthma
- Chronic obstructive pulmonary disease (COPD)
- Crohn's disease
- Ulcerative colitis
- Empty nose syndrome (ENS)

Who is this Book Written for?

1. **Any unwell chronic illness sufferer regardless of whether not yet diagnosed, recently diagnosed, or diagnosed for a long time.** In fact, while the undiagnosed may particularly utilize the sections on diagnosis and access to healthcare, the discussions on mental health, stress, grief, and relationships apply more to the recently diagnosed and long-time sufferer.

   Furthermore, while the spiritual content early in the book offers personal insights and several Bible verses – which Christian readers may particularly appreciate – my goal is to inspire *all* chronic illness sufferers, first and foremost. Plus, research shows the benefits of faith to good health, as this is an evidence-based, psychology self-help book.

2. **Loved ones, the well spouse, and caregivers of the chronically ill.** Chapter 7 provides specific guidance on what one should say, what one should not say, and what one could do to help their loved one. It also discusses the important roles of well-spouses and caregivers in the lives of their chronically ill loved one. Often overlooked, their needs matter, too.

3. **Mental health and medical professionals who treat those with chronic illness.** Examples include counselors, psychologists, social workers, psychiatrists, primary care providers, and specialist physicians.

Your Invisible Chronic Illness

Your situation and thoughts are different. A chronically ill person must think about that which the healthy person does not have to, such as their joints, lungs, bowels, back, or nose. By contrast, these body parts on a healthy person will simply continue to operate at full capacity without any conscious thought.

Now, as noted earlier, 96% of chronic medical conditions in the United States are *invisible*, making them both harder to diagnose and for others – family, friends, and healthcare providers – to understand. As a result, because others tend to assume what we can or cannot do simply by how we look, they tend to downplay this suffering and assume we are either lazy, irresponsible, or even faking our illness.

To add insult to injury, some healthcare professionals who do not understand these complex physical conditions may mistakenly view them as psychosomatic – that the mental state of the condition contributed to or caused the actual physical condition.[a] In this respect, they confuse cause and effect, believing the psychological caused the physical condition when it is in fact the other way around.

This is particularly true of conditions that are considered on the edge of medicine. For example, this is how healthcare professionals have traditionally viewed many physical illnesses such as chronic fatigue syndrome (CFS), fibromyalgia, and Lyme disease.

Because of this difficulty in diagnosing and understanding an invisible chronic illness, delay in diagnosis is the norm, particularly for rare or poorly understood diseases. Considering the serious impact these conditions have on quality of life and, if left untreated, the increased potential for organ damage, any delay in diagnosis can have severe negative effects.

───────────⌖───────────

[a] Only a psychiatrist in collaboration with a psychologist can accurately diagnose a somatic disorder. Additionally, the psychiatrist must access all your medical background and interview you. Your primary care provider or specialist cannot diagnose a somatic disorder!

In addition to preoccupying thoughts, misunderstanding from others (including from medical professionals), and delays in diagnosis, one may also deal with self-blame, financial hardship, career and lifestyle limitations, and navigation through a complex medical system. These stressors, in turn, will undoubtedly impact a patient's mental health, with one-third of chronically ill patients experiencing depression.[3b]

It is not hard to imagine how chronic physical illness can cause depression. Chronic illness sufferers must make major life adjustments and usually experience loss of energy, abilities, relationships, and productivity. They have lost the life they once knew; and the more fulfilling life they enjoyed *before* their illness, the more difficult it is to adjust *after* their illness.

This depression, in turn, can exacerbate the physical condition. Depression can prevent the patient from successfully treating the disease and can contribute to additional physical ailments as well. Consequently, the physical illness' adverse impact on emotional well-being creates a vicious, downward cycle.

The good news is that depression is highly treatable. Your thoughts and actions exert a tremendous impact upon your moods, and *Finding Joy* provides clear, targeted advice on how to change them. If that's not enough and you need professional assistance, *Finding Joy* explores various psychotherapies that can help.

But while depression is highly treatable, you still have to navigate life – including relationships and the medical field – and chronic illness can and will turn your world upside down. It's ever-present, relentless, and pernicious. You can try to ignore and deny it exists and attempt to go

---

[b] The rates of mental health disorders – even from high quality sources – are likely underreported, as many chronically ill patients do not want to carry the additional stigma of a mental illness.

about your life as if everything is fine, but not for long. That plan backfires as you don't meet your goals due to the illness-imposed limitations, and your physical symptoms worsen in the process.

Here are four all-too-common scenarios that reflect life with chronic illness:

♦ You were successful in your career but, thanks to your illness, now you find yourself unable to keep up with company expectations, stay as productive as you would like, or even meet basic work goals. In a worst case (but not uncommon) scenario, you can no longer work.

♦ You love your hobbies and they bring you great pleasure, but you can no longer do them as well as you once did – if at all. You no longer have time or energy for them, as you seem to need rest or sleep over living. Your musical talent may be compromised. Your exercise routine may be shortened if you can do one at all. Or you can no longer engage in your favorite sport that once brought you much joy.

♦ You love spending time with family and friends, but now this time with others must be limited as it exhausts you. You may be an extrovert, but now identify more with introverts. Your loved ones don't understand, and they may be critical or judge you, which you then internalize as well. This creates endless tension in relationships and you might wonder who your true friends are and/or why they have disappeared.

♦ On top of keeping up with your career, hobby, socialization, or basic daily responsibilities, your life becomes an endless cycle of doctor appointments, healthcare pursuits, and medical bills. Never mind the doctors who work against you. You can forget about everything else, including spending time with loved ones. Your life is consumed with the medical merry-go-round.

This is heavy stuff. Chronic illness is not just a monkey on your back, it's an 800-pound gorilla! It can ruin your life. It's okay and perfectly normal to feel down when your world crumbles. In fact, it is very important to experience your feelings, however terrible they may be, because denying such feelings almost always backfires as they become more persistent and pronounced. Only by experiencing such feelings can you deal with them, heal, and improve.

Similarly, it is only by recognizing a problem exists that we have taken the first and most important step to finding a solution. While we may not be able to reverse the physical (or even mental health) ailment or even its trajectory if it is progressive, we can control how we respond to it. In so doing, we should try to strike a balance between being too controlling or obsessed and too defeated or complacent. Easier said than done, we must aim to manage our illness and our mindset in an intentional, focused manner without letting it control our lives.

I get it. Change is hard. Your life is upside down and you might only be able to make small changes in your life after reading this book. But making small or even tiny changes, over time, leads to big results. After all, it is not always the situation in life that determines your well-being, but how you *respond* to the circumstances. Likewise, your response to hardship, no matter how small or seemingly insignificant, can make a real difference in your life.

Now let me ask you: Do you feel mostly at peace with or burdened by your chronic illness? Are there areas in your chronic illness journey that you could improve? Do you want to live your best life despite the challenges and confines of chronic illness?

I know I personally struggle to implement the strategies in this book, but I am determined to never give up and I celebrate the small successes. With even small changes, the benefits are worth it. I challenge you to adopt the same mindset.

How to Apply the Strategies

Key considerations for applying the strategies in *Finding Joy* include:

1. **Keep it simple.** Simple gets done. Select one or two strategies and work on them faithfully over time so that they become habits and part of your daily life.

2. **Be realistic.** These strategies will not cure your physical ailment, some are palliative in nature such as stress reduction techniques, and others will take time to see results. Plus, what helps one person might not work for the next.

3. **Choose what section(s) to read based on your current situation.** Don't feel like you have to read this book in order. For example, if you feel depressed, you might not be ready to tackle the mental shifts suggested in chapter 1. Go straight to chapter 4 which is on grief and loss. If stress is high in your life, go to chapter 3 which discusses ways to reduce stress. If your relationships have been going downhill, go to chapters 5 or 6. If you are a loved one or caregiver, go to chapter 7. If you are struggling with diagnostic or prognostic uncertainty and/or having difficulty navigating the medical field, go to chapters 8 and 9. Want a few diet tips? Go to chapter 10.

4. **All strategies are tailored to chronic illness.** Examples include pacing, exercise considerations, and work at-home possibilities.

   Ultimately, it is up to you as to how you implement the strategies. Use your personal judgement and don't overdo it. For example, if you know you need several days to rest and recover from a large social gathering or outing, then avoid it or make alternative plans if you can.

Me and My Illness

I am blessed to have a family and the ability to work as a school psychologist, which are two realities that I realize not everyone with chronic illness has. But like most with chronic illness, I incur daily hidden struggles. I experience chronic fatigue, breathing difficulties, and I have a demanding physical ailment that consumes hours each day just to manage properly. Consequently, I practice pacing daily in order to not overdo it. In fact, I personally identify best with those who suffer most – particularly the severely debilitated – as our symptoms and experiences with navigating the medical field are often strikingly similar.

Further, I understand the self-blame, relationship impacts, and difficulty accessing high quality medical care all too well. My conditions continue to be challenging in my life. Yet because of good medical care, extensive self-educating, a supportive family, and most importantly, striving to follow the principles set forth in this book, I have effectively managed my invisible chronic illnesses. Although far from cured, I feel joy and gratitude in my life – and I am confident that my mental health is facilitating enhanced physical health.

As a school psychologist, chronic illness sufferer, and Christian, I integrate my personal and professional perspective while backing up associated claims of efficacy with an evaluation of the scientific research. I personally believe that my faith and science go hand in hand, with science showing me how God works. While the central emphasis in this book is integrating positive psychology with communicating, thinking, feeling, and behavioral approaches, it would be incomplete to share what is beneficial for coping, but deny the spiritual aspects of my journey. I do not want to leave you hanging.

There is one caveat, however, as an overly rosy portrayal of a chronically ill patient can be misleading and blatantly dishonest, like someone trying to show off their perfect life on Facebook or Instagram, while tucking away the skeletons in their closet: my chronic illness can, and often does, creep up at *any moment* and rob me of my energy and physical health. When this happens, it does not mean that the medical field has failed me, I am not a positive person, or I do not understand key strategies for good health. It simply means that I have a chronic illness.

Yet after 25 years of dealing with multiple disabling chronic illnesses, I have learned much along the way, I have reasons for much hope, and I am pleased to explore and examine those key elements – on a personal and professional level – that have uplifted me from deep discouragement or despair to living with a sense of purpose, peace, and joy. I trust they can do the same for you.

As the great American Theologian Albert Barnes said: "We can always find something to be thankful for, and there are reasons we ought to be thankful for even those dispensations which appear dark and frowning." Unique and unprecedented opportunities and silver linings abound in dark times, and that could not be truer when it comes to living with a chronic illness.

Chapter 1

Best Psychological Strategies for Chronic Illness

Practical Tips

- ✓ Accept Your Illness
- ✓ Show Self-Compassion
- ✓ Use Positive Reappraisal
- ✓ Apply Positive Self-Talk
- ✓ Adopt an Internal Locus of Control
- ✓ Practice Pacing
- ✓ Celebrate the Baby Steps
- ✓ Expect "Roller Coaster" Progress

Accept your Illness

As an inevitable part of the human experience, everyone experiences suffering and pain in life. Everyone also experiences difficult thoughts and feelings in life. When faced with unpleasant realities, we instinctively try to avoid them by either not thinking about them or trying not to feel them, by analyzing and/or rationalizing them, and/or by outright denying them. These attempts to avoid or deny such thoughts or feelings backfire, however, as such thoughts or feelings almost always become even more pronounced and persistent.

Conversely, we must confront our thoughts and feelings. After all, how we respond to these difficult recurring thoughts or feelings can change the trajectory of our entire lives – for better or worse. We can lead a life moving toward prosperity, fulfillment, and contribution or one toward pathology and hopelessness. In the same way, how we respond to the difficult thoughts and feelings that a chronic illness will inevitably elicit can determine how we view our illness (as a gift or burden), how effectively we manage it, and how we move forward in many areas of life. We can move that trajectory of life needle either upwards or downwards.

Acceptance offers an incredibly powerful step that means to recognize an illness or reality for what it is – without any value judgment. Acceptance does not mean endorsement or approval of it, that you are "okay with what has happened," nor does it mean resignation or giving up. Rather, acceptance empowers you to live freely in accordance with your reality and to find peace no matter your circumstances. When you fully accept your condition, you can truly move forward.

Fully accepting your invisible chronic illness can take a long time, sometimes *years*. It can be difficult to accept our condition because of a lack of diagnosis, conflicting medical opinions, inconsistent, changing health experiences, inner denial or, most likely, a combination of these factors. And when we do reach this point of acceptance, we may accept our condition much better at some times than others, as we move along and between the different stages of grief. Additionally, even for those who have fully accepted their condition, it can still remain a constant balance in thinking between acceptance for a condition as is and hope for better health or fewer symptoms.

Despite an immune deficiency disorder diagnosis in 2008, I did not accept it until 2014. In addition to the standard medical treatments of antibiotics and nasal steroid sprays for sinus infections, I attempted to manage them with every remedy I could try, including surgical interventions. I hoped the rate of my sinus infections would decrease with each remedy I tried, and sometimes they did – for a period of time. More often than not, however, they returned with a vengeance. I had high hopes that my 2009 sinus surgery would "fix" my relentless sinus infections. While it corrected the recirculation phenomenon and I felt thankful for this surgery, my sinus infections continued. In 2010, at age 30, I underwent a tonsillectomy. This reduced my rate and severity of sore throats, for which I also felt thankful, but my sinus infections continued relentlessly. In the meantime, I tried numerous supplements, exercise routines, weekly allergy injections, acupuncture, and nutritional and herbal strategies. Yet my sinus infections persisted. My attempts to control the sinus infections were ultimately futile, as I had not yet accepted my immune deficiency disorder. I was in denial, and this denial prevented me from accessing the help I needed.

I accepted my immune deficiency disorder in 2014 and began receiving direct treatment for it. In 2014, I moved forward.

So aim to accept your chronic illness. Despite the clear limitations your invisible chronic illness imposes, you can still live a life of abundance. By accepting your invisible chronic illness, you can now align your goals and objectives in life with the reality of your illness – and meet them!

A Christian Example of Acceptance

Christians accept the reality of our sinful nature and that faith in Christ saves us from our sins. We cannot change our sinful nature and become sinless, a frustrating and futile endeavor. We cannot measure up to God's standards, nor earn our way to Heaven through good works. In acceptance of our sinful nature, however, we can pray, ask for forgiveness, read the Bible, and make daily decisions that will facilitate a closer relationship with Christ.

In short, by accepting our sinful nature and need for Christ, we are free to live out our faith accordingly. My sister once had a bumper sticker on her car that read: "Christians aren't perfect, just forgiven." This sums it up perfectly. In fact, this bumper sticker caught my wife's attention the first day I met her!

A Christian Example of Acceptance (cont.)

The Apostle Paul accepted his life circumstances and remained not only at peace with adversity, but also highly productive while imprisoned – by authoring 13 books of the Bible! Despite enduring so much adversity, Paul wrote in Philippians 4:11 & 13 (NIV): "...I have learned to be content whatever the circumstances" and "I can do all things through Christ who strengthens me." Far easier said than done, we need to aim for a similar mindset of contentedness and acceptance in living with our chronic illness.

Acceptance and Commitment Therapy

Acceptance and commitment therapy (ACT), an evidence-based therapy considered a third wave of cognitive behavior therapy, could help many with chronic illness. Psychologist Steven Hayes, PhD, developed ACT in 1982. It uses acceptance, mindfulness, commitment, and behavioral change to help patients clarify their values and lead a more fulfilling life. In so doing, the patient improves psychological flexibility – which means to stay present in the moment despite painful thoughts or emotions, and to change or persist in behavior based on the situation and one's values.

ACT includes six main processes, as follows:

1. **Acceptance:** We accept unpleasant experiences as they occur, without attempting to change or deny them.

2. **Cognitive defusion:** As we face negative experiences, we create space between us and our thoughts and feelings – letting them come and go rather than being immersed in them – so we do not fixate on them as much. We reframe our thoughts and see the bigger picture.

3. **Being present:** We stay present and fully aware of our circumstances and experiences, without placing judgment on them or trying to change them in the moment.

4. **Self as context:** We are not merely the sum of our experiences, thoughts, or emotions – what happens to us – but we are the ones experiencing them.

5. **Values:** We engage in those activities that give our life meaning.

6. **Committed action:** We commit or take action toward our goals in a way that is consistent with our values.

ACT offers an effective treatment strategy for many chronic illnesses, such as the management of chronic pain. One study showed that ACT helps in decreasing depression and pain intensity, and improves physical functioning and quality of life.[1] And unlike other treatment modalities that attempt to eliminate chronic pain as the main objective, ACT seeks to allow a chronic pain sufferer to be more active and functional without necessarily eliminating the pain. The patient learns to accept unpleasant experiences and negative thoughts and feelings instead of trying to fight against them. The patient stays grounded in the present, and does not constantly try to figure out how to minimize their pain. By not getting wrapped up in negative thoughts and feelings, such thoughts and feelings can no longer bully behavior.

Show Self-Compassion

A chronic illness provides a constant reminder to self-blame, which leads to decreased self-esteem and depression. We blame ourselves for overdoing it, for needing extra rest, for our "decrepit" bodies, for falling behind at work, for failing to socialize, and for not accomplishing our daily activities or striving toward long-term goals and dreams. To add insult to injury, when we voice this self-blame, our seemingly "able-bodied" friends and family members may also inadvertently join in the criticism either by what they say, by what they do, or by encouraging us to act beyond our physical limitations. This destructive cycle of negative self-regard must not only be stopped, but also reversed, in order to effectively manage our chronic illness.

Self-compassion offers the best way to stop this cycle of negative self-regard. Self-compassion holds a positive self-view and regards oneself with kindness during times of trouble. Among patients with chronic illness, self-compassion leads to lower stress levels, better emotional regulation, better adaptive coping skills, and improved health practices.[2] Psychologically, it promotes happiness, conscientiousness, optimism, and decreases depression and rumination – thinking the same thought over and over without an end or solution.[3]

Three Key Features to Self-Compassion

Psychologist Kristin Neff, PhD, proposes three key features to self-compassion: self-kindness, common humanity, and mindfulness.[4]

1. **Self-kindness** shows genuine care and sympathy for ourselves in light of our perceived inadequacies, shortcomings, or limitations, and thereby resists the urge to be self-critical. *We accept our imperfections and try to let go of our past mistakes. We recognize our value and unique strengths, gifts, or talents.* We stay gentle toward ourselves when we do not reach our self-imposed ideals. Instead of saying, "I can never get anything done because I am so tired," for example, we could show self-kindness and state, "My body is telling me that I need rest right now so I can have more energy and get more done later."

2. **Common humanity** suggests that difficult experiences are part of the human condition and we all suffer at different points in our lives. It recognizes the universal nature of our suffering.

Making small talk with someone at a store, listening to a friend, or showing empathy for someone who is distressed provide examples of connecting with others. The more connected you remain with other people's experiences, the more you realize everyone suffers in one way or another.

The shared vulnerability experienced during the worldwide coronavirus pandemic of 2020, during which millions were infected and died, offers a unique glimpse into common humanity. During the coronavirus pandemic, a common slogan on television ads was "We are all in this together" in reference to the universal pain and suffering. Many with chronic illnesses felt comfort in knowing of the protections for everyone but especially the most vulnerable through masks to prevent the spread of illness, employers accommodating those with chronic illness by allowing them to work from home or take extra safety precautions at work, and social distancing recommendations which some with chronic illness instinctively practice anyway.

3. **Mindfulness,** according to Dr. Neff, means taking a balanced view of one's negative emotional states rather than becoming embroiled in them. Mindfulness does not attempt to ignore or deny these difficult feelings, but simply acknowledges them for what they are, without exaggerating or suppressing them. Mindfulness stays focused on the present, not stressing about the past or worrying about the future. When we notice ourselves feeling stressed, for example, we just note, "Here is stress." We might also note, "This too shall pass," and so we simply sit with it and breathe. Meditation is an example of mindfulness, and it can be as simple as taking a few deep breaths and freeing your mind of any passing thoughts, or saying a prayer.

> The clock only moves forward.
>
> Do not dwell on the past,
> or worry about the future.
>
> Today is enough.

Use Positive Reappraisal

Look at a situation differently. See the silver lining. Reframe your negative thoughts into positive ones. After all, our bodies react to perceived stress, not the actual stress, as two people may react to the same chronic illness in a very different way. Furthermore, you may not be able to change your chronic illness, but you can change how you see your chronic illness. Just as binoculars alter what we see, from far away to close up so we, too, can change how we view our chronic illness by thinking about it differently.

Psychologists define this process of reframing as positive reappraisal. Through positive reappraisal, we respond to stressful situations by attempting to re-interpret them as harmless, valuable, instructive, and useful. As an emotional regulation strategy, our positive thoughts lead to increasingly positive emotions. Positive reappraisal does not mean avoiding all negative thoughts and feelings, but simply changing them into positives. Positive reappraisal is associated with improved moods, reduced distress, emotional resilience, adaptive coping, optimism, happiness, joy, gratitude, and hope.

Do note: Chronic illness can absolutely be very limiting and restrictive in many aspects of our lives, from socialization to physical activities to pursuing occupational or personal hopes and dreams. Our lives can feel that much more limited. Yet by thinking about chronic illness differently, we start to realize the opportunities that a chronic illness presents. As a result of our chronic illness, we might meet new people we would have otherwise not met, appreciate even more those physical activities we can still participate in, not take anything for granted, or pursue an occupation and/or hobby we would have otherwise not discovered.

Despite the clear limitations a chronic illness imposes, how we think about it matters – not only for our moods, but also for our physical health.

Examples of Positive Reappraisal

"Chronic illness serves as a constant reminder of my sickness."

TO

"Chronic illness acts as a *built-in reminder to take care of my health.*"

"Chronic illness led to lost relationships and many judgmental people who I thought were my friends."

TO

"Chronic illness *created new friendships with people whom I share a special bond and unique experience.*"

"Chronic illness forces me to lose control over so much."

TO

"Chronic illness forces me to *recognize what I do have control over, while being at peace with that which I don't.*"

"Chronic illness caused me to lose so much time and positive life experiences."

TO

"Chronic illness has given me a *much deeper appreciation in life in all aspects — for the time I am here and all of my life experiences…*

I do not take anything for granted.
I do not sweat the small stuff.
I am just thankful to be alive."

A Popular Reframe

When life gives you lemons, make lemonade.

Negative reappraisal, similar to positive reappraisal, involves reframing an event, but it reframes it as less negative. For example, instead of thinking how you do not have the energy to make dinner and wash dishes, you remind yourself that you may not seem to have the energy but at least you can wash dishes because you have clean running water, soap, and a sink.

Apply Positive Self-Talk

Self-talk is that continuous internal dialogue that leads our inner voice to send messages to ourselves on a constant basis. We all do it. Self-talk stems from conscious and unconscious beliefs, and from our views about the world and ourselves. These messages range from kind, encouraging, and supportive to critical, distressing, and destructive.

Research shows that positive self-talk results in reduced stress, more confidence, more emotional resilience, and less depression and anxiety.[5]

We humans have a tendency toward negative self-talk. This is particularly true for those of us with an invisible chronic illness, as our symptoms and our acceptance of our chronic illness ebbs and flows. Negative, critical self-talk causes shame, self-absorption, and inaction, while positive self-talk calms fears and improves confidence.

Five common negative self-talk statements among patients with chronic illness include:

1. "Why me? What did I do to deserve this?"

2. "I am a failure. I cannot do that."

3. "I want to be normal."

4. "Look at how little I did today."

5. "I am unlovable."

Brené Brown, PhD, LMSW, a research professor at the University of Houston, describes these negative voices in her head as "gremlins." In so doing, she distances herself from her thoughts, and pokes fun of them. Viewing our self-talk in the third person makes our thoughts seem less personal and easier to change.

Now let's re-look at those "gremlins" from above and change them:

1. Let's change "Why me?" to *'What's next?'* You did nothing to deserve a chronic illness. It just happened. Rather than seeing yourself as a victim of circumstance, you bravely conquer the next challenge – with incredible courage, deep strength, and an incisive perspective.

2. Let's change "I am a failure" to *'I marvel at how much I accomplish.'* Even getting out of a bed is a big deal. A chronic illness imposes limitations and accomplishing even small tasks is dignifying.

3. Let's change "I want to be normal" to *'I will tackle the 'new normal,' whatever that might be.'* As Forrest Gump said, "What's normal, anyways?"

4. Let's change "Look at how little I did today" to *'My batteries just needed re-charging.'*

5. Let's change "I am unlovable" to *'I am worthy of love and respect, and I accept myself and my chronic illness for who I am and what I have.'*

Three Tips for Stopping Negative Self-talk in its Tracks

1. Catch yourself the second you notice your negative thought stream.

2. Replace negative thoughts with positive ones by reminding yourself of your good qualities and prior experiences.

3. Stop comparing yourself to others, as no one wins in the game of comparison, although downward social comparison – comparing ourselves to those we think of as less fortunate – can make us feel better about ourselves in the moment. Nevertheless, I would remind you of the proverb, "comparison is the root of all inferiority."

Adopt an Internal Locus of Control

Psychologist Julian Rotter, PhD, first introduced the concept of locus of control in 1954. Two types of locus of control are internal and external. An internal locus of control refers to the belief in one's ability to control the environment, events, and outcomes, while an external locus of control refers to the belief that we have no control over our environment and life's circumstances that come our way; rather, outside forces, circumstances, and the environment control us. When you are confronted with a challenge in your life, do you feel that you have control over the outcome? If so, then you have an internal locus of control, and that can definitely work to your benefit in managing your chronic illness.

Research shows that people who use an internal locus of control report lower levels of stress and fewer physical problems.[6]

However, because of the suffering and subsequent tendencies toward self-blame and negative self-talk, some with chronic illness tend to apply an external locus of control. As a result, they become much more attuned to what they *cannot* change than what they *can* change. This belief system, in turn, can lead to inaction.

On the other hand, as a result of losing some degree of control over their health, other patients with chronic illness may try to exert even more control over their lives than the average person. In an endless pursuit of better health, first they try to control their health and all aspects of it. When they recognize they cannot fully control their health, their control needs may meander to non-health related aspects of their lives that appear more controllable, such as money, careers, or even relationships.

Yet simply believing we can control our environment may not be enough for managing chronic illness. We also need self-efficacy, the belief that our actions will produce the desired outcome. Good self-efficacy requires thoroughly understanding our conditions and the treatment protocols, accessing and maintaining high quality healthcare, and receiving support from others, whether from family, friends, online communities, or patient organizations. Additionally, while an internal locus of control generally results in better health outcomes, taking an external locus of control on those aspects of our health that we absolutely cannot change could be helpful, as we accept our condition for what it is.

Ultimately, most people adhere to some mix of an internal and external locus of control in their lives. That's why understanding the difference between what we can and cannot control is key to taking control of, and total responsibility for, our health.

The age-old advice to focus on what we can do in the present, not what we cannot do or to dwell on past mistakes, seems fitting. The Protestant Theologian Reinhold Niebuhr wrote the well-known serenity prayer, which is recited at the beginning and end of Alcoholics Anonymous meetings and other 12-step groups. It offers an excellent framework on how we can manage our chronic illness and lives in general. It highlights that we need to accept our chronic illness for what it is, attempt to change what we can in our management of it, and to understand the difference between what we can and cannot change.

Serenity Prayer

God, grant me the serenity to accept the things I cannot change,

courage to change the things I can,

and the wisdom to know the difference.

Practice Pacing

Don't overdo it. Very little must absolutely get done today. We are particularly prone to overdoing it when we are feeling at our best and not thinking about our physical limitations and needs.

Pacing, a popular concept among chronically ill patients, means not overdoing our activities which can make our symptoms much worse. Two types of pacing exist: symptom-contingent pacing, not overdoing it based on our symptoms; and time-contingent pacing, not overdoing it by scheduling in timed breaks.

Pacing results in fewer "crashes" and a decrease in symptoms. Conversely, when we overexert ourselves, we take two steps forward, but often three or more steps backward as our symptoms worsen and we need that much more rest.

The Push/Crash Cycle

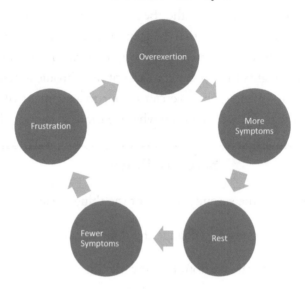

Rather than a "no pain, no gain" mentality, pacing requires spacing out activities and alternating between activities and rest so you can ultimately accomplish what you can without exacerbating your symptoms. Think of Aesop's fable, "The Tortoise and the Hare." Although the tortoise proceeds at a slow pace throughout the race and the hare starts out fast, the tortoise eventually crosses the finishes line first as the hare essentially pushed and crashed. The same phenomenon happens with chronic illness.

Research shows pacing effectively reduces fatigue and increases energy levels among chronic fatigue syndrome (CFS) patients, for example.[7]

The energy envelope theory – a management system that incorporates pacing – states that we need to stay within our available energy or else we will suffer from post-exertional malaise or payback by overextending ourselves.

Within the energy envelope, we have three items:

1. Our available energy: the energy we have to accomplish things.

2. Our expended energy: the energy already used up from physical and mental exertion.

3. Our symptoms: examples include brain fog, fatigue, and pain. When we expend more energy than we have available, we have stepped "outside our envelope" and our symptoms worsen and increase.

A similar theory called the spoon theory, developed by award-winning Author and Speaker Christine Miserandino, started from an effort for her to explain lupus to her friend; lupus is an autoimmune condition that causes inflammation of various body parts. The spoon theory states that the spoons represent a unit of energy and those with chronic illness use up our spoons – and deplete our energy reserves – very quickly. Marbles in a bowl or tokens have also been suggested as other ideas for representing energy units.

Five Tips on how to Practice Pacing for Chronic Illness

1. **Develop a schedule for what you hope to do each day.** Keep the list short with prioritizing of tasks. Additionally, a draining task, which can adversely impact your ability to get other tasks accomplished, might be planned *later in the day* so that it does not prevent you from getting other tasks done, as it can easily drain an overwhelming amount of your energy. You can use Google Tasks to create a short to-do list, and you might wish to use a timer so you can keep on track with your schedule.

   You can also develop a schedule through a daily planner. You can list your tasks or activities and categorize them into "high priority," "medium priority," and "low priority." Examples might include emailing, texting, phoning, or face-timing a friend; cleaning or decluttering specific rooms; and ordering items online or buying them at a store. When you deem a task a low or medium priority, you know you have additional days to complete this task and that relieves some of the self-imposed stress. Plus, projects and large tasks often take two to three times as long to finish than what we initially anticipate. And technically, much in life does not need to be completed in one day.

Expect that your daily schedule will deviate from your planned schedule due to interruptions and the unexpected. This will happen and it presents the greatest deterrent from implementing pacing. Do not give up at this point. Simply revise your schedule. In his song, *Beautiful Boy*, the famous Musician John Lennon sang, "Life is what happens to you while you're busy making other plans."

Additionally, if you face an unexpected stressor such as a tense encounter, a surprise bill, or a cumbersome, lengthy meeting, you might find that you will not be able to accomplish *anything* further that day. That's okay.

2. **Plan for scheduled rests and/or take frequent breaks in your daily routine.** After a period of activity, a break might include lying down for 10 minutes, reading your favorite book, or taking a walk. If you take a nap during the day, it is better to do it early in the day or before 2:00 so that it does not interfere with your sleep. Some patients recommend the use of a heart rate monitor such as a Fitbit watch to keep track of how you are doing and to rest when you notice your body needs it or, better yet, *before* your body needs it.

If working, you may need to be creative about where to take this break and it may need to be shorter than 10 minutes, as your employer will frown upon this if visible. In these instances, closing your eyes at your private work area, resting in your vehicle during a break, or relaxing in a private locked room during your lunch break can provide a few moments of respite.

3. **Know your limits.** While self-explanatory, our invisible chronic illness symptoms change constantly, with ebbs and flows. You need to listen to what your body tells you and adjust accordingly. If you know an activity might push you over the edge, don't do it.

4. **Slow down when doing tasks and do them right the first time.** You do not need to do everything very fast nor everything at once. And if you rush a task and do it incorrectly, then you will most likely spend more time fixing it than you would have if you had proceeded more slowly and carefully in the first place. Just like the tortoise and the hare story proves, slow and steady wins the race.

5. **Aim to use 75% of your available energy and thereby accomplish about 75% of your scheduled activities.** This approach, although perhaps difficult to come to terms with for the overachiever, ensures a safe level of activity. For example, rather than attempting to reorganize the entire garage, take satisfaction in reorganizing half or three quarters of the garage. By keeping your expectations at this level, you can better pace yourself and prevent the push and crash cycle. Some of us perfectionists and over-achievers particularly need to heed this advice.

Celebrate the Baby Steps

The late Actor Hugh Beaumont played the role of an epitomized suburban father, Ward Cleaver, in the popular television sitcom comedy

Leave it to Beaver. My own family enjoys watching *Leave it to Beaver* on a regular basis 60 years later. According to Hugh's daughter, Kristan Beaumont, he remarked that to change anything, "You need to start small." He noted that you cannot accomplish everything at once. "You start by tying your shoes."[8] Hugh clearly appreciated the importance of baby steps in reaching big goals.

Financial guru and Talk Show Host Dave Ramsey developed a system of baby steps on the path to financial freedom. His first three baby steps, which must be followed in chronological order, involve building a starter emergency fund, paying off all debt (except your mortgage), and then building a three-to-six-month emergency fund. His last four baby steps, which do not need to be followed in an exact order, involve investing for retirement, saving for your children's college, paying off your mortgage, building wealth, and becoming what Dave calls "outrageously generous."

Clearly, staying focused and investing your energy toward one thing often provides the means to much larger success later on. Where you focus is where you win. This principle seems true in many areas of life. For those with chronic illness, this means taking that first baby step and then cherishing each baby step along the way in our management of chronic illness.

Such baby steps help us to more effectively manage our physical limitations, as we improve our physical health while accepting its limitations.

For example, now that I know how nebulized saline can improve my bronchial hygiene, my bronchiectasis might improve a little as well. Baby steps also help us to overcome perceived barriers to improved physical health. Now that I know my bronchiectasis can improve a bit, I can now aim for higher goals with respect to bronchiectasis, such as an additional reduction in symptoms. All goals, big or small, start with baby steps.

Lastly, once you have identified your personal or health goal you want to work toward, write it down. Writing down your goals makes them clear and objective, and increases the likelihood you will achieve them, as it serves as a reminder and helps you stay focused and motivated.

Expect "Roller Coaster" Progress

When it comes to chronic illness, progress is not linear and often fluctuates up and down on a continuous basis with flare-ups, improvements, and occasionally new symptoms. This unpredictable aspect of living with a chronic illness forces us to constantly adapt to the changes.

On that note, it's important to bear in mind that sometimes treatments help only a little. Over time, however, this little bit of help eventually adds up to a lot of help. So try to be patient with your health as you endure this marathon.

For example, since developing bronchiectasis in recent years, my rate of sleep apnea (repeated cessation of breathing when asleep) has become increasingly inconsistent, despite the daily use of a humidified continuous positive airway pressure (CPAP) device. This is because the mucus in my sinuses will travel downward toward my lungs as I sleep, leading to buildup. Because of bronchiectasis – which involves difficulty moving and coughing up phlegm – lower respiratory breathing becomes increasingly difficult as the night progresses. Yet some nights I can sleep 7 to 8 hours with low rates of sleep apnea. Other nights, I struggle to obtain 5 or 6 hours of sleep with higher rates of sleep apnea.

Nevertheless, as I increasingly learn how to better manage my bronchiectasis, my sleep has slowly and gradually improved, although it still feels like being on a "roller coaster" at times!

In this respect, perhaps it could be argued that progress of a chronic illness should be measured in *years*, not days. This is similar to that age old question we might ask ourselves after we have seen that same healthcare professional for a year: "Are you better off or worse off than when you first started seeing your healthcare provider?"

Chapter 2

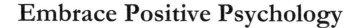

Embrace Positive Psychology

(While Understanding its Limitations)

T he field of positive psychology, with Psychologist Martin Seligman, PhD, as its father, incorporates individual character strengths, virtues, and behaviors to build a life of meaning, purpose, and deep satisfaction – the good life. In so doing, positive psychology empowers individuals to not merely survive, but to flourish.

My employer implements a school-based program at the elementary school called The Positivity Project or P2.[c] This program is based on positive psychology and the work of positive psychology co-founder, Christopher Peterson, PhD. It includes lessons, assemblies, and announcements to teach character strengths – such as integrity, gratitude, fairness, honesty, and humor – as well as an "other people matter" mindset to become more self-aware and empathetic, and to build positive relationships. Given positive psychology's focus on how we relate to and treat others, at the end of the morning announcements the speaker will say, "Hashtag," and everyone enthusiastically replies: "Other people matter!" Character traits such as those just mentioned along with a focus on serving, helping, and encouraging others provide the foundation for positive psychology. In the same way, we may not only encourage others, but in the process improve ourselves, whether healthy or living with an invisible chronic illness.

An abundance of research reveals that positive psychological traits – such as good moods, optimism, life satisfaction, and purpose – promote good mental and physical health.[1] For example, a long-term

[c] West Point graduates and Iraq and Afghanistan veterans Mike Erwin and Jeff Bryan founded The Positivity Project in 2015.

study on nuns revealed that the nuns who were the happiest lived on average 10 years longer than the least happy nuns.[2] Positive psychology has clearly made an invaluable contribution to both our collective mental and physical health.

Positive psychology also goes hand in hand with psychoneuroimmunology (PNI). Robert Ader, PhD, coined the term psychoneuroimmunology in 1980, a field which investigates how our minds and emotional states directly impact our immune system. Dr. Ader's contributions include our understanding of the immune response to stress and illness, as well as the power of the placebo effect.[d]

For further reading on how our minds can impact our physical health, two excellent books are *Biology of Belief* by Bruce Lipton, PhD, and *How Your Mind Can Heal Your Body* by David Hamilton, PhD.

Positive psychology, however, will not cure your chronic illness. In fact, a systematic review on positive psychology and chronic illness revealed its beneficial impact on moods, quality of life, and pro-health behaviors, per se, but that its direct impact on a chronic physical health ailment remains largely inconclusive and requires further study.[3]

Does this mean you should abandon positive psychology in striving to improve your invisible chronic illness? Absolutely not! As just noted, much research shows positive psychology does significantly contribute to physical health and longevity among healthy subjects. Armed with this knowledge, it seems logical to conclude that positive psychology also contributes to enhanced physical health among those with chronic

---

[d] Dr. Ader founded the journal Brain, Behavior and Immunity, and was the founder and past president of the Psychoneuroiummunology Research Society. Dr. Ader was a professor emeritus of Psychiatry at the University of Rochester Medical Center. He also served as past president of the Academy of Behavioral Medicine Research and the American Psychosomatic Society.

A placebo is that which represents medical treatment, but has no therapeutic value; rather it is based off a patient's perceptions or expectations.

illness, as a mind and body approach seems ideal for managing chronic illness. Just stay realistic on its limitations.

Because *Finding Joy* already covers many considerations that fall under the umbrella of positive psychology such as acceptance, self-compassion, reappraisal, positive self-talk, locus of control, pacing, and social support, this chapter examines how other areas of positive psychology can also enhance your well-being. Specifically, positive psychology is broken up into good thoughts, good emotions, and good behaviors, using well-researched examples for each category.

Before diving into how positive thoughts and emotions can enhance your well-being, it is important to note that you should expect problems to occur in life and recognize that difficult thoughts and emotions are simply a part of life. The good news is that difficult thoughts and tough emotions are usually fleeting and momentary, as they constantly change throughout the day, week, month, and year. We may feel sad at one point in the day, but happy at a different point. What bothers us terribly one day may not be given much more than a fleeting thought the following day. So when you face those difficult times and moments, you can take comfort in the proverb: "This too shall pass."

Positive Thoughts

Embrace Optimism while Understanding the Merits of Defensive Pessimism

While optimism may be thought of as taking an overly rosy view, researchers define optimism as anticipating a favorable future with more positive than negative events. Using this definition, optimists remain realistic about challenges and difficulties, but focus on and acknowledge the positive. Much of the research on optimism, done largely on patients with heart disease and cancer, shows that optimistic and hopeful patients enjoy a high quality of life and satisfaction, take a proactive approach to their health, and their optimism is associated with positive health outcomes and fewer negative changes to their chronic illness.[4]

However, correlation does not imply causation, and further research is needed to determine the exact relationship between optimism and health as it pertains to chronic illness. For example, it cannot be determined if the optimism itself contributed to improved health outcomes, or if the optimism led to proactive behaviors, resulting in better health. Nevertheless, optimism is associated with improved health outcomes of a chronic illness.

In the 1980s, Psychologist Nancy Cantor, PhD, proposed an alternate view to optimism and the "don't worry, be happy" mindset so ingrained in American culture, which she called defensive pessimism. By anticipating negative events and scenarios and setting low expectations for your performance, defensive pessimists can prepare for and avoid these obstacles in pursuit of their performance goals. It should be noted that defensive pessimism is not a global style of thinking, but rather an approach to meeting specific goals. In *The Positive Power of Negative Thinking: Using Defensive Pessimism to Harness Anxiety and Perform at Your Peak*, Psychologist Julie Norem, PhD, argued that positive thinking does not adequately address the pressures and anxieties in modern life. She presented case examples of highly successful defensive pessimists.

As it pertains to chronic illness, I believe the value of defensive pessimism is limited to the context of a recurring, specific negative health challenge. For example, one may anticipate their acute health crisis or progressive chronic illness to worsen unless they take proactive measures for their health. However, because of the negative thinking and extra focus on what can go wrong, defensive pessimism is associated with higher levels of trait anxiety and low self-esteem.[5-6]

A personal example of how defensive pessimism can apply to chronic illness is when I incur a sinus infection. I could try to stay upbeat and optimistic that the infection will resolve without medical intervention but, because of my immune deficiency and a weak nasal defense system, I am aware that my sinus infections rarely resolve without antibiotics. By anticipating that the worst will occur, I can take action by contacting my physician who will take a culture and prescribe an antibiotic, thereby eradicating the infection.

Find Meaning and Purpose in Suffering

Living life with meaning and purpose positively impacts your psychological and physical health. An Ohsaki, Japan study of 43,391 adults revealed that those who lived a "life worth living" ("ikigai" in Japanese) were significantly more likely to be alive seven years later than those who did not.[7]

I have found incredible meaning and purpose from living with my invisible chronic illness. While my search for better health never ceases, I view this suffering as a part of life from which I can grow and learn.

Confronting these chronic illnesses on a constant basis has changed my worldview and caused me to become more grateful, more humble, more kindhearted, more eager to help others, and more reliant on God. No matter the level of suffering, *I am always seeking the reason behind it.* The reason might not be apparent in the moment, but it might be to bring people together, to give me a break, to modify my treatment plan, to grant me new insight into a problem, or to offer me an even deeper appreciation for when my suffering is milder.

Below are 10 examples demonstrating how my chronic illnesses have increased my meaning and purpose in life:

1. My invisible chronic illnesses have strengthened my faith in God. I believe God has a purpose behind all my suffering. I rely on God for assistance in my weakness and I view the suffering here on earth as short compared to the joy in Heaven.

2. Continuous suffering, while it has caused too much self-focus, has also cultivated a humble, nonjudgmental, kindhearted attitude in me. I do not have the time, energy, or motivation to act any other way.

3. I am grateful for each day of life and do not take anything for granted. I want to live each day to the fullest.

4. I am grateful for my wife and children, for their patience with me as I spend two to three hours daily treating my health through nasal washes, nebulized saline, inhalers, use of a high frequency chest wall oscillation vest, and infusions with immune globulin.

5. I am grateful for the many friends with chronic illness whom I have met on my journey, as well as for the exchange of ideas in our shared experiences. Invisible chronic illnesses allow me to connect with others who also suffer on a deep level.

6. I am grateful for the opportunity to use my strengths in helping others with chronic illness. I can help others with similar conditions through my writing, my words, and my actions.

7. I am grateful for the healthcare professionals whom have taken their time to listen to me, have problem solved and offered

potential solutions, and have granted me access to high quality healthcare.

8. I am grateful for access to treatments which effectively manage these conditions. The advancements in modern medicine are incredible.

9. I am grateful for the little things – a smile or encouraging word, a helping hand, or the birds eating from birdhouses – that others take for granted.

10. I am grateful for access to nutritious food and clean water.

To further explore your life purpose in living with a chronic illness, *Finding Purpose: Rediscovering Meaning in a Life with Chronic Illness* provides an excellent springboard.

Stay Open to New Experiences

Staying open to new experiences – such as trying a new hobby, learning new skills, or keeping an open mind to fresh ideas – is positively associated with good physical health.[8] Those open to new experiences tend to adapt well to change be it in their career, life circumstances, or relationships. Those open to new experiences tend to be creative, inquisitive, adventuresome, and intellectual. However, we tend to be less open and more routine-oriented as we age.

An example of openness is my desire to learn and apply new information about bronchiectasis. Because I have an unquenchable thirst for knowledge in understanding and in treating bronchiectasis, which has wreaked havoc on my sleep, I comb through research on best practices for its management, inquire with physicians, and willingly try new treatments. For example, I learned that N-acetyl cysteine (NAC) acts as a mucolytic (dissolves mucus), and one study showed that NAC at 600 mg, two times per day, over the course of one year resulted in a significant decrease in bronchiectasis exacerbations.[9] Consequently, I purchased and have been using this supplement.

Stay Conscientious

Conscientious refers to the tendency to be careful, responsible, hard-working, and goal-oriented. A conscientious person does their personal best. They persevere in life, follow the rules, and tend to be high achievers in work and in life in general, with detailed plans to meet their goals. The University of Minnesota Professor and Psychologist William Schofield, PhD, described this person with the acronym YAVIS, which stands for "young, attractive, verbal, intelligent, successful." He noted that many psychologists would prefer to counsel this type of client given the opportunity for therapeutic success.

Conscientiousness is considered a major predictor of health, quality of life, and longevity. It should not come as a surprise then that conscientious individuals with chronic illness have good adherence to their medication regimen and better health outcomes with their chronic illness.[10-11]

Positive Emotions

Humor

In 1964, Journalist and Professor Norman Cousins, PhD, was diagnosed with a crippling and degenerative condition called ankylosing spondylitis, which causes long-term inflammation of the joints and spine. He was in severe pain, with paralysis of his neck, legs, and back. His doctor and friend gave him only a few months to live and a one in 500 chance of recovery. Determined to defy the odds, Cousins took massive doses of intravenous vitamin C and watched numerous comedy shows such as *Candid Camera*, *Laurel and Hardy*, and the *Marx Brothers*. Cousins claimed that 10 minutes of belly laughter offered him two hours of pain-free sleep. Although there was debate whether he truly had ankylosing spondylitis or an acute attack of an arthritic condition, remarkably he recovered from his condition. In 1979, he chronicled his experience with this illness and laughter therapy in *Anatomy of an Illness as Perceived by the Patient*. His story was made into a movie in 1984 and he earned over 50 honorary doctorate degrees. His efforts resulted in the Norman Cousins Center for Psychoneuroimmunology at the University of California, Los Angeles.

Dr. Cousins' story was instrumental in encouraging patients to take a proactive role in their health and it highlighted the importance of the mind-body connection, specifically that laughter offers a great coping tool for dealing with physical hardship. Laughter releases endorphins – hormones referred to as your body's "natural painkillers" – which increase oxygen intake, aid blood circulation, and boost pleasure. As a result, laughter can induce relaxation and thereby decrease your stress, improve your immune system, and improve your mood.[12-16] Consequently, chronic illness sufferers in general and chronic pain sufferers in particular could benefit from a good belly laugh.

In addition to laughter therapy, which includes group or individual sessions to literally show you how to "laugh your stress away," other means for laughing include:

♦ **Watch a funny show, movie, or YouTube video.**

♦ **Read the comics.**

♦ **Laugh at yourself.** Take notice of those awkward moments, or your mistakes or shortcomings, and chuckle about them. If you are like me, you have plenty.

For example, one of my closest and longest friendships to this day started when I told the church congregation to "wait" during a 2nd grade communion speech – as if the congregation would just stand up and impatiently walk out! Embarrassed at the time, little did I realize this incident would lead to a lifelong friendship as we laughed incessantly while watching the video.

Another example is during the receiving line of our wedding, my wife and I both called one gentleman the wrong name ("Bruce" instead of "Garth") based on his proximity to someone else who had a husband named Bruce. We should have known better. He probably had a complex. We still laugh about it to this day.

♦ **Do something peculiar.**

♦ **Laugh about something that you otherwise take very seriously or is even upsetting to you.** For example, if you suffer from arthritis, say "arthritis" as you laugh. It might seem odd and is odd, but it works by helping your body to take a different reaction to the stressor.

Interestingly, you can induce a laugh, which generates the same physical effects as a genuine laugh. This is called laughter yoga. First you breathe deeply through your diaphragm, which is just below your ribs. Then inhale through your nose to a count of four and then exhale through your mouth to a count of four. As you exhale, release a big belly laugh. Repeat this cycle as many times as you wish. You will notice that, after you have induced this laugh, laughing becomes easier and more automatic.

Just know the right time to laugh. Laughing at a funeral or at someone else's expense, rather than along with someone, will not likely facilitate good relationships, thereby affecting your social support.

You can also fake laugh to fit in when you do not understand a joke and wait for your brain to catch up, as the average person can make a fake laugh sound genuine. However, a fake laugh can also backfire, such as when you laugh at someone's expense.

Research into laughing for improving mental and physical health seems very promising, and remains an excellent tool for the chronically ill. Given its often serious and harmful impact, we can take our illness too seriously. It might very well be true that "laughter is the best medicine."

Gratitude

Gratitude is an emotion and attitude of thankfulness. It is a "count your blessings" mindset.

Research shows that gratitude is linked with happiness, and it appears to improve some aspects of physical health in healthy subjects, such as sleep quality.[17] Similarly, one study on chronic illness patients with IBD and arthritis found that increased gratitude was associated with a substantial decrease in depression.[18]

Gratitude interventions are simple and easy to implement. Examples of such interventions include:

- Write a letter to someone whom you have never thanked before. You can also do this by phone.

- Write one thing for which you are grateful each day, or three things each week.

- Write about your best possible self. This is where you envision your life in the future, and write down the strengths or positive character traits you need to reach your goals.

- Give thanks in prayer.

- Stay present in the moment and be thankful for the smells, the sights, or anything else for which you feel thankful.

◆ Write in a gratitude journal.

I have occasionally kept a gratitude journal and I would like to share part of my entries from early 2020:

> I am thankful that my in-laws watch our children so my wife and I can go on monthly date nights. I am also thankful that our children are getting older, so our older children can watch our younger children for date nights as well.

> I appreciated how our neighbors invited us to sing Christmas carols with them to the neighbors on our road.

> After a planning meeting for Stockade – a 3rd through 6th grade boys ministry for which I volunteer – the leader gave us a bottle of pure maple syrup.

> I am thankful to have access to treatments for bronchiectasis.

> Despite being awake until 3:00 AM the prior night because of a massive storm, my neighbor came over early the next day and assisted us in cleaning up a small tree that had fallen on our property.

Happiness

Before discussing happiness, it is important to distinguish between happiness and joy. While a simple Google search of "define joy" reveals "a feeling of great pleasure and happiness" and the terms are sometimes used interchangeably, they generally have different meanings to most people. Joy is construed as a stronger emotion than happiness, an internal attitude that is ever present and sacred, while happiness is construed as a fleeting emotion based on an end destination, goals met, or external events. I personally view joy and happiness as going hand in hand because if you experience joy – although you will not always be in a state of happiness – an inner, lasting sense of happiness will likely follow.

Optimistic and grateful people tend to be happier than pessimists. Happiness is associated with many positive physical health outcomes among healthy people such as lower stress, stronger immunity, reduced blood pressure, more rapid healing, and increased longevity.[2, 12-14]

Happier people who have chronic illness employ better self-management by not only attending to their medical needs, but also by staying socially connected, eating well, and exercising. For example, one study showed that patients with rheumatoid arthritis who were happier reportedly experienced less pain and fewer symptoms than those who were less happy.[15] It should be noted, however, that this does not prove the subjects in fact incurred less pain, but rather that they reported and perceived less pain.

An extremely important point: to suggest that you should just "not worry, be happy" is disingenuous, as it ignores the fact that health itself plays a large role, an even larger role than our wealth, toward our levels of happiness. As discussed earlier, chronic illness is associated with high rates of depression. *And the more disruptive your chronic illness to your everyday functioning, the more depressed you tend to be. This helps explain why some with very serious medical conditions such as cancer might be happier than those who have less threatening, but long-term, disruptive conditions such as urinary incontinence and rheumatoid arthritis.*[16] Because your chronic illness itself can lead to depression, you may need cognitive behavior therapy, self-talk strategies, and social support, to name a few, in your pursuit of happiness.

Happiness, however, can be an elusive state of mind that we strive for as most people find themselves ranging between the highs and lows of everyday life.

If interested in learning about what the science says makes us happy, Psychology Professor and Head of Silliman College at Yale University, Laurie Santos, PhD, teaches a popular course called *Psychology and the Good Life*. This course provides tips for making wise choices in life so we can lead a happier, more fulfilling life. This course dives deep into the question: "What makes people happy?" And what makes us happy *may not be what you think,* as people react to the meaning they attach rather than the event or circumstances themselves.

You can listen to many of Dr. Santos' lectures and interviews on her podcast, The Happiness Lab. For example, by listening to her podcast I have learned that:

◆ Winning the lottery can sometimes be the worst thing to happen to someone.

◆ Despite their convenience, ATM machines and their lack of human interaction adversely affect happiness.

◆ Too many options at a restaurant can lead to information overload and unhappiness.

Love

Love is a strong feeling or deep affection we have for something or someone. By showing love to others, we show others we deeply care about them and value their relationships. We are close to such people. This love that comes from a marriage relationship, family, or strong friendships serves as an important source of emotional and social support during a chronic illness. And social support serves as a strong protective factor for chronic illness. Those in committed relationships, for example, experience less stress, better healing, show healthier behaviors, display a greater sense of purpose, and enjoy a longer life.[20]

Examples of love include:

- ◆ Acts of kindness.

- ◆ Helping another person in their time of need.

- ◆ Listening.

- ◆ Doing an activity even when you do not feel like doing it.

- ◆ Putting your loved one's needs first.

- ◆ Romantic interest.

Love is a particularly important concept in Christianity. In Matthew 22:37-39, Jesus states that the most important commandment is to love the Lord your God with all your heart, soul, and mind, and the second most important commandment is to love your neighbor as yourself. In Ephesians 5:25 (NIV), the Apostle Paul states that husbands should "love their wives just as Christ loved the church and gave His life for it."

For those who want to strengthen their marriage or for those whose marriages may be struggling, *The Love Dare* is a book with an accompanying movie, *Fireproof*, which includes a 40-day challenge for demonstrating unconditional love. Each day you read a key idea, perform a love dare, and journal your thoughts. Like any relationship, building a healthy marriage requires time, effort, and a lot of love.

Furthermore, in his #1 *New York Times* bestseller, *The 5 Love Languages: The Secret to Love that Lasts*, Pastor and Marriage Counselor Gary Chapman, PhD, helps you fine-tune your preferred methods for giving and receiving love. I learned these love languages while dating my now-wife Colleen, and putting them into practice has enhanced our relationship.

The five love languages are:

1. **Words of affirmation:** Be specific and elaborate on what you appreciate about your loved one. Saying "I really appreciate how you speak so calmly and lovingly with our children" is an example of words of affirmation. This is my wife's love language.

2. **Acts of Service:** Show your love through action. Examples of acts of service may be sweeping and mopping the floors, or better yet, making a dinner for your loved one. This is my love language.

3. **Quality time:** Provide your loved one with your time and undivided attention. This is also my wife's love language.

4. **Giving gifts:** Give your loved one a present, small or big.

5. **Physical touch:** This touch may include a pat on the shoulder or a hug, and it is not to be confused with physical intimacy.

Positive Behaviors

Embrace Your Faith

The viewpoint through which we see the world has a profound impact in how we respond to trials and tribulations. As a Christian, I have great hope in my eternal destination and I view the suffering here on earth as small in comparison to an eternity in Heaven. In many respects, my faith in Jesus helps me to make sense of suffering, as it provides clarity and purpose to it. Without this faith and clearly defined purpose, my suffering would lead to increased hopelessness and despair.

As an acronym, a Christian might argue that "joy" stands for "Jesus first, yourself last, and others in between." There is even a song that accompanies this fitting acronym.

Spirituality

I consider myself both religious and spiritual. While religious and spiritual are terms used interchangeably and that often go hand in hand, a religious person is commonly, but not always spiritual, while a spiritual person may or may not be religious. I am religious in that my set of beliefs include that Christ died to save us from our sins, and that I try to live a lifestyle that is based on a set of morals and values as found in the Bible. I am also spiritual in that, in addition to my belief system and activities associated with my religious faith, I attach meaning and purpose to that which affects my spirit or soul.

An abundance of research reveals that increased religiosity and spirituality is associated with improved health outcomes, better coping skills, a higher quality of life, less depression, and greater meaning, comfort, and hope among those with chronic illness.[21] The literature does not differentiate the effectiveness between different religions, however. Rather, the literature views religion and spirituality as enhancing methods – such as through social support or engaging in healthy behaviors, for example – to improve health, while also noting they add a dimension of meaning and purpose to the suffering. By adding purpose, they reduce some of the anxiety and uncertainty associated with chronic illness.

Forgiveness

I believe that Christ forgives those who accept him as their Savior. Likewise, I believe that I need to forgive others who I perceive have wronged me, and to ask for forgiveness of those whom I have wronged.

The concept of forgiveness, defined as acknowledging fault and, in turn, letting go of negative feelings often in regard to interpersonal conflict, is associated with numerous health benefits: reduced risk of a heart attack, reduced blood pressure, increased immune system, improved relationships, improved sleep, and decreased anxiety, stress, and depression.[22-23]

Forgiveness does not guarantee that you will reconcile your relationship with others, nor does it guarantee the other person will change. It does not excuse or forget the harm done or approve or allow of the bad behavior; you still need to set boundaries.

Rather, forgiveness allows you to live with greater peace, happiness, and joy, freeing yourself from the clutches of anger, bitterness, and hurt. You let go of such negative feelings and condemnation – you let go of the past – which makes it much easier to show compassion and empathy to others and to *yourself*, and this ultimately leads to better spiritual and physical health.

Prayer

Religious and spiritual people often pray. I pray and I have seen in my own life that God answers prayer.

However, prayer and meditation, terms used interchangeably, are different. Meditation usually involves decreased thinking, or removing "the chatter in your mind," while prayer involves talking to God, for example, and praying for forgiveness, healing, and striving to maintain a closer relationship with God.

While the research does not examine whether God answers prayer, per se, it shows a host of health benefits associated with prayer: improved mood, lowered stress, reduced blood pressure, better sleep, improved cognitive functioning, shorter and fewer hospital stays, and increased longevity.[24-25] So prayer may benefit not only those you pray for, but yourself as well!

Volunteer

Research shows that staying productive if not altruistic (selfless concern for the well-being of others), particularly in our areas of strength – be it through volunteer, academic, or professional work – leads to reduced stress, increased happiness, improved cognitive skills, greater social connectedness, and increased longevity, as long as the work being done does not overwhelm.[26]

Volunteering shifts our thoughts from ourselves to others and, in so doing, gives us a greater purpose, improved self-esteem, and increased life satisfaction. We take an other-orientation and, in the process, help ourselves. For example, I wrote a monthly newsletter for the International Empty Nose Syndrome Association for two years, 2016 and 2017, and it felt fulfilling to not only disseminate current news on ENS to others and use my writing skills in the process, but also to stay connected with other ENS sufferers.

Various nonprofit organizations exist that allow people to stay productive. In retirement, my father-in-law, for example, assisted with driving the elderly to medical appointments or to the grocery store, as well as with a local organization that offers horse rides for children with disabilities.

Other volunteer opportunities include:

♦ Maintaining a local park.

♦ Assisting at a food pantry or soup kitchen.

♦ Reading to children at a local school.

♦ Helping at an animal rescue shelter, art museum, or library.

♦ Offering professional services for free.

If going out and about places too much stress on you because of pain or the limitations imposed by your chronic illness, you can also volunteer from home. For example, moderating an online community forum of a chronic disease, sharing your experiences with others or psychologically supporting others, or using your technology skills, are just a few volunteer opportunities you can do from home.

Engage in Lifelong Learning

Learning is a lifelong, cumulative process, often self-initiated and resulting in personal growth. Countless opportunities for learning exist, both in-person and online. This learning often requires staying open to learning new skills and fresh ideas. Such learning does not stop when we finish college, trade school, or other types of formal education.

Lifelong learning is associated with overall improved health outcomes for those with chronic illness. Keeping your mind active improves your sense of purpose, self-efficacy, self-esteem, thinking skills, social networking, and emotional resilience – adapting to crises or stressors.[27] What you spend time learning about, however, should be relevant and address your interests, strengths or gifts, and/or needs. For example, I enjoy learning about various practices that promote good health, reading the Bible, and I would like to learn how to play the drums.

Chapter 3

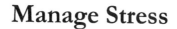

Manage Stress

S tress is a normal, everyday part of life – and how you manage it has profound implications for your health. Broadly defined, stress refers to the emotional strain or physical tension we experience in response to a stressor such as a challenge, demand, or pressure. Types of stressors include relationships, jobs, significant life events, and physical health. While some types of short-term stress are benign or helpful, chronic, negative emotional stress is regarded as a "silent killer" as it is a major contributing factor to the leading causes of death in the United States.[1]

Your chronic illness represents a major life stressor in and of itself, contributing to your overall stress level. And it is the failure to recognize just how much stress you are under that represents a serious threat to your health. While you cannot eliminate stress, your chronic illness and the hustle and bustle of everyday life and resulting constant stress can normalize dangerous stress levels. Consequently, strategies to reduce stress from your chronic illness and manage stress in general remain of paramount importance.

Most strategies contained in *Finding Joy* can reduce your stress levels. By increasing your resilience to stress through thinking and behavioral strategies, by practicing a healthy diet and exercising as you are able, by nurturing good relationships, and by engaging in the stress reduction methods in this chapter, you can reduce flare-ups, prevent disease progression, and enhance your overall health. Plus, your stress load will be lower so you can better handle other stressors when they do come your way.

Five Types of Stress

1. **Distress:** negative stress. Types of distress include suffering, pain, anxiety, worry, guilt, discomfort, and trouble. An example of distress is feeling guilty for not having the energy to complete a household task.
2. **Eustress:** positive or beneficial stress. This stress makes life exciting, such as skiing down a mountain, going to a party, or for some, preparing for a speech. It is important to note, however, that the body does not differentiate between eustress or distress, as too much of a good thing can also cause wear and tear.
3. **Acute stress:** short-lived stress. An acute stressor for someone with a chronic illness is a flare-up of your chronic illness, such as increased pain.
4. **Episodic stress:** frequent bouts of acute stress. The effect of multiple bouts of stress is cumulative.
5. **Chronic stress:** long-term stress. This is what can feel overwhelming or beyond what we can handle.

General Adaptation Syndrome

Hans Selye, MD, PhD, regarded as the "father of stress research," was an endocrinologist who studied the physiological response to perceived stress.

From his research, he proposed the general adaptation syndrome (GAS), which includes three bodily stages of adaptation in response to stress:

1. **The alarm stage:** This first stage includes your body's "fight or flight response" and initial physiological symptoms such as an increased heart rate, increased release of cortisol (stress hormone), and increased adrenaline.

2. **The resistance stage:** This stage occurs after your body has adjusted to the initial shock. While your body attempts to adapt and repair itself, it remains on high alert and continues to secrete a high level of stress hormones. You may also have high blood pressure in this stage.

3. **The exhaustion stage:** This third and final stage follows after the resistant stage continues for too long and depletes too many bodily reserves. The exhaustion stage results from prolonged or chronic stress, and it places your body at high risk for harm, including the development and/or progression of chronic illnesses.

Given the long-term or indefinite nature of a chronic illness, you can easily find yourself in the exhaustion stage, thereby causing your chronic illness to worsen in a seemingly endless vicious cycle. As a result, implementing stress-reducing techniques is critical. So in addition to the various strategies discussed elsewhere in *Finding Joy* that can reduce stress, chapter 3 explores numerous stress-reducing techniques such as mindfulness, meditation, fun, and more.

Mindfulness

Mindfulness, the opposite of forgetfulness and a popular technique which involves training our minds to be present, is a promising stress reduction technique for the chronically ill. While we tend to think our minds are focused on the present, our minds often wander to dwell on the past or worry about the future. Our minds race with a lot of chatter. More than an attempt to merely free us from distraction, mindfulness reduces the power of those distractions.

Three key mindfulness skills are:

1. **Observing:** This is noticing what is going on around or within you without judgment. Imagine you just had a difficult encounter with a family member who made critical comments toward you. You observe feeling angry by the hurtful comment, but you attempt to stay detached from this anger and not act upon this feeling. You identify the emotion and try to avoid an emotional reaction; rather, you simply notice what is occurring. In this respect, observing helps you to know yourself better.

2. **Describing:** This is labeling what occurred without judgment. For example, in describing how you responded to the hurtful encounter, you might note, "I struggled to respond calmly when my spouse raised his voice."

3. **Participating:** This means staying present and fully engaged with the activity. For example, after the difficult encounter occurred and the dust settled, you accurately and clearly expressed to your spouse how these comments made you feel and you gave your full attention to his point of view as well.

It should also be noted that, although often used interchangeably, mindfulness and meditation are different terms. Mindfulness focuses on staying present, while meditation is an umbrella term that means to achieve a highly focused state of mind with complete self-regulation of your mind. In this respect, mindfulness can essentially be a form of meditation.

Research shows that engaging in mindfulness is associated with a host of health enhancing benefits including reduced stress, better sleep, lower blood pressure, lower body mass index, less pain, stronger cognitive performance, and better attention.[2-3]

I have attended many mindfulness seminars in my career. Five recurring mindfulness activities include:

1. **Release of tension:** You tense and relax your muscles, and then observe your body as it becomes increasingly relaxed.

2. **Simple breathing exercises:** You direct attention to your breathing as you inhale and exhale, noticing each breath.

3. **A quiet moment:** You are still. This might involve closing your eyes, dimming the lights, and simply hearing sounds, listening to relaxing music, or noticing a pleasant scent.

4. **Guided visual imagery:** You visualize yourself in a different setting. For example, you picture yourself at a beach with the sun warming your skin, the light breeze moving through the air, and the sound of waves crashing gently in the ocean.

5. **Loving kindness activity:** You express kindness to yourself or to a loved one, with thoughts such as "May he/she feel happy and be doing well, healthy to whatever degree he/ she can be, and may he/she be protected from harm."

Breathing Exercises

Problematic breathing of the chronically ill may result from a lower respiratory ailment, such as chronic obstructive pulmonary disease (COPD) or an upper respiratory ailment, such as chronic sinusitis or empty nose syndrome.

A normal resting breathing pattern should involve breathing primarily through the nose and driven by the diaphragm rather than through the mouth and driven by the upper chest, shoulders, or neck, the latter of which typify breathing disorders. Whereas healthy breathing is constant, rhythmic, quiet, and automatic, unhealthy breathing is shallow and quick. Consequently, those with unhealthy breathing patterns essentially need retraining on how to breathe. Attempting to normalize these unconscious breathing patterns through breathing retraining leads to overall improvements in lung functioning, a relaxation response, and stress reduction.[4-6]

While many types of breathing techniques exist to improve your breathing, the basic premise behind most breathing exercises is to slow your pace of breathing and make it more efficient by increasing oxygen intake into, and by removing carbon dioxide out of, your lungs. By slowing down your breathing rate, they keep your airways open longer, remove trapped air in your lungs, and temporarily decrease shortness of breath.

Four breathing exercises are:

1. **Diaphragm (also known as abdominal) breathing**

    ♦ Sit or lie down.
    ♦ Put one hand on your stomach and the other hand on your chest.
    ♦ Inhale through your nose for two seconds, and let your belly push your hand out. (During this inhalation, your chest should not move).
    ♦ Exhale through pursed lips for six seconds as if you were blowing out candles. Feel the hand on your belly go in, and use it to push all the air out.
    ♦ Do this breathing exercise up to ten times.

2. **Pursed lip breathing**

    ♦ Sit down.
    ♦ Relax your shoulder and neck muscles.
    ♦ Slowly inhale through your nose (with your mouth closed) for a count of two.

- Pucker or "purse" your lips, as if you are going to blow out a candle.
- Then exhale through pursed lips for a count of four.
- Repeat this cycle until you normalize your breathing.

3. **4-7-8 diaphragm breathing, as recommended by Dr. Andrew Weil**

- Sit or lie down.
- With your mouth closed, inhale through your nose to a count of four.
- Hold your breath for seven seconds.
- Exhale through your mouth for eight seconds.
- Repeat this cycle four times.

4. **Alternate nostril breathing**

- Sit down and cross your legs.
- Place your left hand on your left thigh.
- Close your right nostril with your right thumb.
- Inhale through your left nostril.
- Then close your left nostril with your right thumb, and exhale through your right nostril.
- Inhale through your right nostril.
- Then close your right nostril with your right thumb, and exhale through your left nostril.
- This completes one cycle.
- Repeat up to five times.

A popular breathing method known as the Buteyko method was developed over four decades, beginning in 1952. The Buteyko method offers seven different techniques specifically tailored to the adult or child's needs, and it addresses conditions such as nasal congestion, sleep apnea, asthma, stress, anxiety, and panic attacks.

The Buteyko method also includes a controlled pause – which involves holding your breath after inhalation – and it encourages your tongue to rest on the roof of your mouth, which encourages correct tongue posture and promotes nasal breathing.

You can learn more about the Buteyko method by visiting the Buteyko Clinic's website or by watching its YouTube videos.

To learn more about breathing techniques, two excellent resources are *The Wim Hof Method: Activate Your Full Human Potential* and *Breath: The New Science of a Lost Art*.

Exercise

Exercise in any form is an effective stress reducer. By engaging in exercise, your body produces endorphins, improves your mood, enhances your physical health, and reduces stress. Ultimately, your exercise routine should include some combination of aerobic exercise, strength training, and stretching.

It can be very difficult, however, for the chronically ill to engage in an exercise routine or even walk because of frequent health flare-ups and/or mobility issues. I can personally attest to this fact, as I would often incur sinus infections shortly after attempting an aerobic exercise routine. In a 2018 study, subjects with chronic fatigue syndrome who engaged in minimal exercises took several days to recover from the post-exertional malaise – i.e., symptom flare-ups and substantial energy crashes.[7] These failed attempts and setbacks are discouraging. Consequently, certain considerations should be taken into account for exercising with a chronic illness.

Exercise Considerations for those with Chronic Illness

1. **Only exercise when your body can handle it.** A moderate or severe flare-up is a sign not to exercise, or to only engage in light exercise.

2. **Do only what you are up for doing.** You may need to decrease the amount of time or intensity of your exercise, particularly when you are experiencing a mild flare-up of symptoms.

3. **Start with light exercises.** Examples include a short walk, light stretching, or lifting a lightweight dumbbell.

4. **Select exercises that will not cause flare-ups.** If you experience low back pain, for example, you may need to consider swimming or walking rather than tennis or running.

5. **Select fun exercises.** Select exercises that you enjoy doing which helps with motivation.

6. **Pair your exercise with another enjoyable activity.** For example, while you go for a jog, you may listen to music or to your favorite speaker. If you prefer to socialize while exercising, find a friend to exercise with.

7. **Talk with your doctor about what exercises are safe for you.** Your doctor may conduct a medical exam or a stress test to help guide this determination.

8. **Mix up your exercise routines to keep them interesting.**

9. **Take enough time, perhaps even days, to rest and recover.**

10. **Build an exercise routine into your daily schedule as much as possible.** Determine the time of day, amount of time, and specific exercises. Attempt to fit in exercise, even brief exercise, if you have a very busy schedule.

Interval Training

Interval training mixes exercise intensity in a workout, allowing you to pace yourself. Given the need for pacing, interval training exercise may be a wise choice for those with chronic illness. One example of an interval training exercise is jogging or brisk walking for three minutes and then normal walking for one minute, and repeating this pattern for 15 minutes. When I am feeling up to it, I personally enjoy a similar exercise routine on my elliptical.

As you may be aware, research has shown that high-intensity interval training (HIIT) exercise reaps some of the same benefits as moderate intensity exercise in a mere fraction of the time. An example of a simple, brief, and effective high-intensity interval training exercise is the "nitric oxide dump." As the name implies, it releases nitric oxide throughout your body, thereby slowing down the aging of your muscles and improving blood flow. Originally developed by Physician Zach Bush, MD, it involves 160 movements, it takes 2 to 3 minutes, and it may be done up to 3 times per day. The four components of the nitric oxide dump include 10 or 15 repetitions of 1) a squat; 2) a circular arm swing; 3) a static forward march; and 4) a shoulder press.

You can watch chiropractor Dr. Joe of Dr. Joe TV demonstrate how to complete a nitric oxide dump and/or Natural Medicine Physician Dr. Joseph Mercola's demonstration video.

Yoga

Yoga involves stretching, coordination, and balancing activities, and it incorporates breathing, meditation, and exercise. In fact, Jon Kabat-Zinn, PhD, developed a technique of combining meditation with mindfulness and yoga called mindfulness-based stress reduction (MBSR).

As most commonly practiced, yoga usually involves various physical postures, which improves strength and endurance, improves cognition, increases focus, and in turn reduces stress and improves overall well-being. Specifically, yoga has been shown to increase overall functioning, increase the immune system, and decrease stress among people with chronic illness.[8] People with chronic illness can particularly benefit from yoga because you can adapt the intensity of yoga to how you feel each day, from rigorous to gentle and restorative. You can do it daily at your pace and intensity.

You may be able to find local public classes that teach you how to get started with yoga, although it might make just as much sense to start through private or online instruction. Consider starting with gentle and restorative yoga, if possible. Websites such as Yoga Journal, Glo, and Gaia offer various resources including online instruction, articles, and videos.

Nature-Based Activities

Most people spend much of their time indoors, with a tendency to spend even more time indoors as they become adults. Yet spending time outdoors is associated with increased movement and exercise as well as various health benefits, including increased happiness and vitamin D resulting from the light exposure, increased concentration, increased creativity, increased compassion to yourself and others, and reduced stress.[9] While countless outdoor activities exist, three common outdoor activities include grounding, taking a walk, and gardening.

Grounding

Grounding, also known as earthing, involves having skin contact with the earth such as walking barefoot on the grass. Grounding is based on the premise that connecting to the earth's natural energy is the foundation for optimal health. Our bodies have electrical energy. As a result of electromagnetic radiation, particularly from mobile phones and

Wi-Fi, for example, our bodies have a lot of positive electrons. These positive electrons in the form of free radicals can then be balanced out via a negative grounding charge. Grounding results in improvement with inflammation, sleep, blood pressure, pain, and stress.[10]

In recent years, I purchased a grounding mat from Amazon for under $60 so I could do grounding from the comfort of my home during the winter months when skin contact with the earth was not feasible. I was concerned with the amount of electromagnetic radiation exposure due to the amount of time I spent on my computer at home and work, as well as radiation from my smartphone.

For more information on grounding, read *Earthing: The Most Important Health Discovery Ever!*

Walking

If you are able and feel up to it, walking outside in the fresh air is a potent stress reducer. Walk outside each day and your stress level will tank in no time. Walking is an easier-to-do activity than running, and it results in less trauma to our knees and bodies. You can do a brisk walk, normal walk, or a combination of the two. If you find your chronic illness is in a state of remission, you can even combine walking with running. Additionally, changing the location and scenery of where you walk can keep your walk interesting as "variety is the spice of life." If you are fortunate to live near a mountain or lake, for example, you could hike up the mountain or around the lake.

Three additional tips to consider when walking:

1. You should stretch before and after your walk to prevent injury to your leg muscles.

2. Start small by walking for 10 or 15 minutes before building up to 30 minutes.

3. If you incur pain with walking, you might want to:

    ♦ Take pain medication before your walk.

    ♦ Massage your leg muscles or use a heat pad or take a warm shower before you walk to increase blood circulation.

    ♦ Apply an ice pack after your walk to reduce swelling.

    ♦ Rather than push through it, if the pain is too much, take a break.

Gardening

Gardening offers another nature-based, health promoting activity that most people can participate in on some level, including the young and old alike, as well as those living with chronic illness. Once your garden is planted, the primary upkeep of it includes watering although it also needs weeding, particularly at the start of the season.

Health benefits resulting from gardening include improved mental, physical, and social health such as enhanced cognition, increased moods, decreased depression, reduced anxiety and stress, as well as increased hand strength and dexterity, improved heart health, weight loss, and increased social connectedness.[11] Not to mention, you get to eat fresh vegetables!

Five basic tips to consider when gardening with a chronic illness are:

1. **Start with a small garden and low maintenance plants that you plan to eat.** You can always add more plants later, but starting small with low maintenance plants makes gardening less time-consuming, more achievable, and it prevents waste.

2. **Take basic outdoor precautions such as wearing gloves.** Those with an immune deficiency disorder, for example, are more apt to get an infection from dirt bacteria.

3. **Start with a raised bed if you can afford it.** Raised beds require less bending and have fewer weeds than a ground-level garden.

4. **Consider purchasing accommodating tools.** Examples include a fold-up stool, garden shovels with comfortable grips, a coiled garden hose, weed cutters that require no bending, and a wagon. Many of these user-friendly tools require minimum bending, and consequently result in less stress on your body and joints.

5. **Limit your gardening to the coolest hours of the day**. Examples include the early morning or late evening hours.

Journaling

Therapeutic journaling, defined as writing down our thoughts and feelings about our personal experiences, offers a range of physical and mental health benefits, including decreased depression and reduced post-traumatic stress.[12-15] You can write down your thoughts on a computer or by hand. Therapeutic journaling differs from traditional writing in a diary, the latter of which includes a detailing of events. By expressing our emotions through therapeutic journaling of a traumatic or upsetting experience, for example, we get a deeper understanding of the problem, of ourselves, and we often gain increased clarity and a new perspective for handling the problem. The therapeutic effect of journaling results from both expressing our emotions and letting go of such feelings.

Social Psychologist and Professor James Pennebaker, PhD, developed an evidence-based, expressive writing protocol used commonly in clinical practice. In this context, therapeutic journaling involves writing for 20 minutes per day for four consecutive days about an upsetting event.

Some key considerations Dr. Pennebaker recommends include:

◆ The event or events should be very personal and important to you.

◆ This should be written just for yourself and shredded afterwards.

◆ You should write continuously without respect to grammar or spelling errors.

◆ You can expect it will increase your emotions, but you should discontinue writing if it elicits too many emotions or is too upsetting. If this happens, you might employ other relaxing activities recommended in this book or, if needed, seek professional help.[16]

I personally have found that journaling about traumatic experiences helps me better cope with and "move on" from them. For example, a recent medical appointment was upsetting to me because of what appeared like a lack of knowledge of my healthcare professional on my medical condition and its implications for treatment. As a result, I wrote about how I felt and listed key points I need to discuss with my healthcare professional. This writing helped me to organize my thoughts for discussion so I can stay focused, move on from the entangling emotions, and it increased my awareness to newfound and various plan B strategies that can address my specific health needs.

As an author, writing this book offers a similar therapeutic effect. I can express all my emotions in dealing with my chronic illnesses, retrieve previously learned psychological concepts and learn new ones along the way, and gain satisfaction from sharing what I know that can be useful.

But journaling is not for everyone. Three examples include someone dealing with severe trauma, someone who has significant difficulty expressing their emotions, or someone who simply dislikes or is unskilled in the writing process, although a speech-to-text technology might accommodate the latter example. In these cases, other options for expressing their feelings might include, but are not limited to: art, music, or dance.

Pleasurable Activities

By planning and implementing fun activities, recreational therapists and assistants have an important job that increases the happiness and reduces the stress of those under their care. Similarly, whatever brings you pleasure should be included or added to part of your plan for coping with chronic illness. Have fun and emphasize experiences over material goods. Because different people have different ideas on what constitutes fun, as one person's fun activity may be stressful for someone else, you need to personalize these activities. Just remember: You still need to pace yourself as too much of a good thing (resulting in "eustress") is still stress and it can overload your system, requiring rest and recovery.

Suzan Jackson, in her practical and helpful book, *Finding a New Normal: Living Your Best Life with Chronic Illness*, poses the question: "What makes you forget [about your chronic illness]?" She cites examples such as drinking tea, looking at the blue sky out of the window, listening to a favorite song, hugging a child, playing an instrument, going for a nature walk, or spending time with a friend or family member. She then encourages the reader to seek more of those moments in their daily lives.

So what brings you pleasure?

- ◆ Fishing
- ◆ Shopping
- ◆ Sunbathing
- ◆ Hiking or walking
- ◆ Watching a movie
- ◆ Birdwatching

- Reading a book or listening to an audiobook
- Swimming in a pool, lake, or ocean
- Attending a sporting event
- Going to a concert or lecture
- Joining a local book club
- Sewing
- Woodworking
- Dining out
- Playing an instrument
- Crocheting
- Cooking
- Hunting
- Going for a scenic drive
- Playing card games, chess, or checkers
- Attending a play or musical
- Doing a puzzle, crossword puzzle, or Sudoku
- Taking a nap
- Martial Arts
- Playing with your pet

Supplements

Supplements appear to work slowly and over time, and I personally take a limited number of supplements with a solid research base. I also share what I am taking with my healthcare professionals to prevent interactions with conventional medicines.

Three supplements which help manage chronic stress are:

1. **Magnesium:** The mineral magnesium helps to regulate over 300 biochemical reactions in the body. It has been referred to as a miracle mineral and the ultimate relaxation mineral with advocates touting its effectiveness in preventing calcification of

arteries, high blood pressure, muscle cramps and spasms, depression, hormone problems, and sleep and energy problems. Personally, I have found that taking 400 mg a day of magnesium citrate (the maximum recommended dose for an adult) has been helpful in relieving temporomandibular joint (TMJ) pain. You can buy it as a tasty powder in a drink from Natural Vitality, or as a capsule.

2. **B vitamins:** These vitamins include eight water-soluble vitamins that improve nervous system functioning and, in turn, reduce overall stress levels. For example, a study of 215 males who took a B complex vitamin for 33 days reported improved health and less stress.[17] I have historically taken B complex vitamins and found they had a relaxation effect.

3. **Herbs:** A Medical News Today article discussed eight herbs that reduce anxiety: ashwaganda, chamomile, valerian, lavender, galphimia glauca, passionflower, kava, and cannabidiol.[18] According to this article, the research showed that most of these herbs exerted some degree of calming effects taken at the right dose, although it also noted cautions and side effects of certain herbs, such as chamomile causing allergic reactions and interacting with blood-thinning medications. Consequently, herbs are a promising avenue for managing stress, particularly if you can research the side effects and be under the supervision of an herbalist. On a personal note, I was under the guidance of an herbalist at one time and found herbs to be helpful.

Simplify

Our lives are complex and even basic tasks and activities include numerous details. Take grocery shopping, for example. Some of the basic steps for grocery shopping include: we get into our car; put the key in the ignition; drive out of the garage or driveway; drive to the store;

stop the car; get out of the car; walk into the store; get a cart or basket; locate groceries on the shelves; bring the groceries to the cash register; pay for the groceries; return to the car; unlock the car; get into the car; put the key in the ignition; drive home; put the car in the driveway or garage; turn off the car; carry the groceries into the house; and finally, put the groceries away. Clearly, these 20 steps can overwhelm! And that's just grocery shopping. We therefore benefit from making our activities of daily living easier to do with the fewest details possible.

Examples of ways in which we can simplify our lives include:

♦ Do a grocery order pickup or, better yet, delivery. Many stores offer these options for free or for a small fee.

♦ Declutter your home or part of it.

♦ Take a break from social media or electronic devices altogether. I admit I am as guilty as anyone for spending too much time on the Internet, but I sleep better without all the blue light before bed, and time away is refreshing and mind-clearing.

♦ Put away your phone during business meetings or social outings.

♦ Avoid toxic people as much as possible.

♦ Say no to more obligations.

♦ Say no to extra meetings.

♦ Dispose of, or better yet, donate those material goods that take up space.

We can also simplify our healthcare routine. For example, I used to spend time doing both nebulized saline as well as steam inhalation to help reduce chest congestion. I eventually removed steam inhalation from my routine, saving myself about 5 minutes each day, as both treatments serve a similar purpose.

Other Stress Relief Options

While stress is a normal part of life, you have abundant options for reducing your overall stress load. Three additional strategies that can effectively reduce your stress load include massage therapy, craniosacral therapy, and a hot bath or Jacuzzi. While you can seek professional services for the first two, you can also implement elements of all three stress-reducing techniques on your own.

Massage Therapy

Massage therapy, defined as patterned and purposeful soft tissue pressing, rubbing, and manipulation, decreases muscle pain and tension, improves sleep, and reduces stress. Chiropractors, physical therapists, and massage therapists are three professions that offer massage therapy. Massage techniques, which can range from light touch to deep pressure, increases the levels of serotonin – a hormone that impacts your mood – and it decreases the stress hormone cortisol.

Three common types of massage therapy are Swedish massage, deep tissue massage, and trigger point massage. Swedish massage includes long strokes, kneading, deep circular movements, and vibration and tapping. Deep tissue massage involves slow and forceful strokes. Trigger point massage consists of direct pressure to sore and tight muscle fibers called knots.

While you can seek professional massage therapy, which I highly recommend, your friend or loved one can also offer you a massage. It may not have the same level of effectiveness as a professional massage, but I am sure many spouses, for instance, find themselves quickly drifting into a deep sleep after a nighttime massage.

Additionally, you can apply deep pressure to your own knots using a Thera Cane, an effective trigger point massager. For additional information on how to self-administer a trigger point massage, read *The Trigger Point Therapy Workbook: Your Self-Treatment Guide for Pain Relief.*

Craniosacral Therapy

Craniosacral therapy is a type of gentle massage therapy that significantly reduces stress. Cerebrospinal fluid pulses like a semi-closed hydraulic system through the entire craniosacral system – the brain and spinal cord – in waves (movements of $1/16^{th}$ to $2/16^{th}$ of an inch) about six to twelve cycles per minute. When these waves become restricted or disrupted due to any number of factors such as an impact, lesion, or strain, symptoms appear.

A craniosacral therapist, who may be licensed in many different specialties such as a physical therapist, chiropractor, or massage therapist, for example, attempts to restore this craniosacral rhythm by gently guiding these craniosacral waves. By restoring these waves, symptoms disappear. A craniosacral therapy session runs from about 30 minutes to an hour. Because of my significant nasal symptoms, I have benefited from craniosacral therapy for the past 12 years.

The most comprehensive option for craniosacral therapy is professional therapy – which insurance often covers if you go to a licensed, practicing professional such as a physical therapist – although you can also apply some of the techniques yourself. For example, you can purchase a Still Point Inducer™ online, which is a simple device that you rest your head on and it pauses your craniosacral rhythm, thereby promoting deep relaxation and less pain. You can also learn and apply some of the craniosacral techniques by reading *Harmonizing Your Craniosacral System: An Easy and Effective Self-Treatment.*

A similar technique to craniosacral therapy, cranial osteopathy is administered by a doctor of osteopathic medicine (DO), with a primary focus on addressing the skull sutures (juncture between the skull bones).

Osteopathic manipulative medicine (OMM), which understands the concept that skull bones move along the sutures, manipulates the musculoskeletal system to treat pain and tension. Pressure in a cranial osteopathy session is more forceful.

A Hot Bath or Jacuzzi

A hot bath or a Jacuzzi offers a free stress reliever with a range of health benefits, including improved blood circulation, reduced blood sugar levels, reduced inflammation, and muscle relaxation.[19] In addition to putting a bath bomb in the tub for your skin, you can also add oils such as rose, lavender, calendula, coconut, or oatmeal. Further, you can add Epsom salt to your bath – a compound of magnesium, sulfur, and oxygen – for added benefit to your sore muscles, your skin, and your digestive tract.

It is important to limit your time in a hot bath or Jacuzzi to ten minutes to avoid overheating and dizziness. Additionally, a Jacuzzi should be cleaned regularly, you should check with your doctor if you have heart disease before immersing in hot water, and pregnant women might need to avoid hot water immersion altogether as the increased body temperature may pose a risk to the developing baby.

Chapter 4

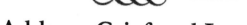

Address Grief and Loss

"Mike," an aspiring young attorney engaged to be married, avidly hiked, played guitar, and remained very active in youth activities. At age 35, his doctors diagnosed him with rheumatoid arthritis, which is a progressive, debilitating chronic inflammatory disease of the joints. While he at first tried to hike at the same rate as before this diagnosis, he soon realized his body was unable to keep up. Additionally, his fingers hurt when he played the guitar and he did not have the energy to remain as active in various youth activities let alone for his profession as an attorney. He experienced great loss in his need to scale back the time put into his profession, his hobbies, and his commitment to the community – the life he once knew. Sadly, realizing the cumbersome nature of his illness, his fiancé called off the engagement. Eventually, despite all he seemed to have going for him, this invisible chronic illness and subsequent loss led to grief, hopelessness, despair, and depression.

The Five Stages of Grief

It is natural and healthy to experience a range of emotions in dealing with chronic illness. Your emotions will range from anger, fear, and frustration to sadness and grief, and all emotions in between. Grief, deep distress or sorrow over loss, seems arguably the most pronounced emotion for a patient with chronic illness.

Most people with chronic illness would say that they have experienced loss such as loss of relationships, loss of a job, loss of time, loss of control over their health, loss of finances, loss of the ability to use their unique talents or passions, and ultimately the loss of plans, aspirations, and dreams for a seemingly brighter future. In short, most chronically ill patients say they have lost a life they once knew. It can seem like being in a fish bowl and seeing the world move forward around you, but you cannot move forward as you remain stuck with your limitations.

While grief is a normal emotional reaction to a major adverse life event – when this grief lasts for a long time, starts to overwhelm, and we cannot function or cope with our loss – it then becomes a problem and we might seek professional help.

The renowned Psychiatrist Elisabeth Kübler-Ross, MD, developed the theory of the five stages of grief, which was based on the range of emotions which terminally ill people experience before their passing, as well as loved ones grieving their loss. These stages offer a framework for what many people experience when dealing with loss. The emotions do not occur in a step-by-step manner, as one may jump around, get stuck in a stage for a long time, or even go in reverse. That's okay and to be expected.

The Five Stages of Grief

1. Denial
2. Anger
3. Bargaining
4. Depression
5. Acceptance

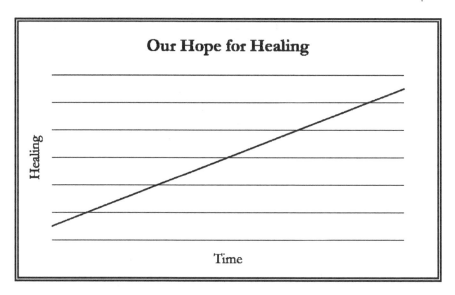

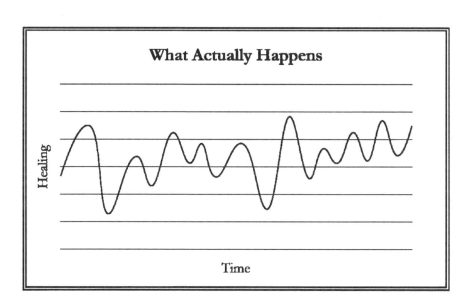

The Seven Stages of Grief (as Adapted to Chronic Illness)

Building upon Dr. Kübler-Ross' grief model, Professor and Counseling Psychologist Jennifer Martin, PsyD, wrote an adaptation to these stages of grief for chronic illness. This new model encompasses the additional stages that her patients who had chronic illness experienced, such as loss of self and confusion and re-evaluation of life, role, and goals. According to Dr. Martin, patients with chronic illness go through these stages in a nonlinear manner, and it sometimes can seem like a continual spiral.

The Seven Stages of Grief

1. Denial
2. Pleading, Bargaining, and Desperation*
3. Anger
4. Anxiety and Depression*
5. Loss of Self and Confusion*
6. Re-evaluation of Life, Role, and Goals*
7. Acceptance

*Represents adaptations to the five stages of grief as proposed by Dr. Martin.

Dr. Martin's seven stages of grief and loss include:

1. **Denial:** The chronically ill patient refuses to acknowledge the chronic illness, and may appear in "shock" and "disbelief." Dr. Martin noted that denial is the most dangerous stage because the patient does not seek the treatment he or she needs.

2. **Pleading, Bargaining, and Desperation:** We may try to do everything we can to return to our "normal way of life" before our chronic illness. Examples include trying to eat super healthy, engaging in rigorous exercise, and doing everything we can to cure ourselves. We may experience a sense of guilt, questioning ourselves, such as "Could I have prevented this condition?" or "Why did this happen to me?" or "How have I deserved this?"

3. **Anger:** Recognizing the permanence of our diagnosis, we feel angry about a lack of cure or treatment options, and/or our newfound physical limitations.

4. **Anxiety and depression:** There tends to be much uncertainty surrounding chronic illness, including its prognosis, when flare-ups will occur, or what the new normal will look like in our daily lives. Such uncertainty leads to anxiety. This uncertainty, compounded by loss and anger, can lead to depression. In fact, anger, anxiety, and sadness often accompany each other. Dr. Martin states these represent normal responses to the uncertainty of our future and a major life-changing event.

5. **Loss of self and confusion:** Given our new limitations, we question our identity and may have even lost part of it. We question our purpose in life, who we are, and how we fit in. We come to terms with our new inabilities, whether unable to perform certain physical activities, activities of daily living, or work-related activities.

6. **Re-evaluation of life, role, and goals:** When determining what we have given up and our purpose in life, we explore new roles and goals in line with our chronic illness and in forming our new identity. Re-evaluation requires flexibility in thinking such as a new career role where we might work from home but do limited hours, or we revisit an old hobby but not overdo it.

7. **Acceptance:** We accept our illness as a new normal, and we have come to terms with the permanency of it. Despite our illness or because of it, we still grow, experience peace and joy, and integrate our chronic illness into our new way of life. We also seek others who help us achieve our goals.

Loss Can Lead to Depression

Extensive loss and the accompanying grief associated with chronic illness can lead to sadness, despair, anxiety, worthlessness, guilt, hopelessness, helplessness, and ultimately depression. As noted previously, about one-third of chronically ill patients also suffer from depression.

Depression, known as the common cold of all mental illnesses, involves persistent sadness, anxiety, pessimism, and helplessness. Depression usually involves a loss of interest or pleasure in previously enjoyed hobbies, withdrawal from social activities, diminished energy, restlessness, irritability, and trouble focusing and making decisions. Depressed patients might experience sleep disruptions, overeating and/or eating unhealthy foods, and persistent physical symptoms. Depression can lead to physical symptoms such as an increased risk of heart disease, pain, insomnia, inflammation, digestive disorders, and weight gain. In the worst case scenario, depression can lead to suicide, which may be thought of as a "long-term solution to a short-term problem." As such, depression can clearly exacerbate a chronic illness.

Thankfully, depression is highly treatable and more than 80% of patients who seek treatment show improvement, yet fewer than half of patients with depression pursue treatment. Clearly, more depressed patients should seek treatment. Treating co-occurring depression usually involves therapy and sometimes medication, or a combination of both. Treating co-occurring depression leads to improved physical health, increased adherence to a medical treatment plan, and an enhanced quality of life.[1]

Additionally, it should be noted that treating the physical condition itself can also lead to less depression. The bottom line: treating both the physical and psychological aspects of a chronic illness will lead to the best health outcome.

Cognitive Behavior Therapy

Cognitive behavior therapy (CBT), an approach that encompasses several specific therapies, remains the gold standard as the most effective form of psychotherapy for treating depression, often getting good results in as few as 5 to 20 sessions. You can be treated online or in person and, if you have insurance, it will often cover it. In fact, I will always remember a professor sharing, during a graduate course on CBT, that research indicates CBT is as effective as medication for treating depression.

CBT posits that our thoughts and feelings are not necessarily due to situations themselves, but our interpretation of them. It focuses on challenging irrational thoughts and negative feelings, which in turn influence our actions and subsequent thoughts and feelings. CBT aims to teach that while we cannot control all our circumstances, we can identify and control our disturbing thought patterns. CBT challenges disturbing thought patterns such as irrational thinking; rumination, dwelling on the same cringe-worthy thoughts over and over; and catastrophizing, believing the worst will happen.

Clinical Psychologist Albert Ellis, PhD, laid the foundation for CBT with rational emotive behavior therapy (REBT). This is a therapeutic approach that posits irrational or self-defeating beliefs regarding life circumstances worsen the problem but – by directly disputing such beliefs and directing the patient to better thinking and behavioral patterns – the patient experiences improved emotional health. Dr. Ellis referred to these irrational thought patterns as "stinkin' thinkin,'" providing examples of irrational thoughts such as overgeneralizing, catastrophizing, self-derogation, an unusually low tolerance for frustration, and rigid, absolutist thinking.

CBT is an action-oriented therapy that uses tools such as reframing, journaling, direct exposure to fear-provoking situations, and role playing. It helps you set and achieve realistic goals in small, manageable steps.

Dialectical Behavior Therapy

Marsha Linehan, PhD, developed dialectical behavior therapy (DBT) in the late 1980s, which is an effective CBT method for depression. Dialectical thinking refers to being able to see issues from opposing perspectives, and attempting to engage in balanced thinking – as opposed to all-or-nothing thinking – by acknowledging that different ideas can co-exist. By fully grasping opposing points of view, DBT asserts one can gradually can gain a closer approximation of the truth.

Dr. Linehan initially developed DBT to address the intense emotions of her patients with suicidal ideation and borderline personality disorder, a disorder which consists of highly unstable moods, behaviors, and interpersonal relationships. This is because her patients were not benefiting enough from CBT, particularly as they found it invalidating. DBT filled in this gap by attempting to understand the context and validate the patient's thoughts, feelings, and actions. By combining validation with a push for change, her patients were more cooperative and the therapy was more effective.

The four primary strategies of DBT are:

1. **Mindfulness:** Mindfulness is a key part of DBT that refers to staying present in the moment, thereby helping you to stay calm. You pay attention to your thoughts and feelings in a nonjudgmental manner by avoiding labeling them as "good" or "bad." Mindfulness, when used in conjunction with CBT

approaches, is called mindfulness-based cognitive behavior therapy (MCBT).

2. **Distress tolerance:** Rather than attempting to change a distressing circumstance, tolerating distress means accepting it for what it is. DBT teaches that acceptance of the circumstance does not mean approval of it.

3. **Emotional regulation:** Many with mood disorders frequently experience intense emotions. Through identification of emotions, building positive experiences, and letting go of emotions or taking the opposite action that would be expected given the current feelings, DBT teaches how to more effectively manage negative emotions and increase positive ones. One such way to identify your thoughts and feelings, as well as coping strategies, is by recording them on a Diary Card and then sharing this card with your therapist at the next session.

4. **Interpersonal effectiveness:** The goal is to build positive relationships by approaching others in a thoughtful and caring manner. DBT teaches the ability to assert your needs and say no to demands when appropriate.

Other Therapies

Additional therapies found to be effective for depression include:

1. **Interpersonal Therapy (IPT):** Psychiatrists Gerald Klerman, MD, and Myrna Weissman, PhD, developed IPT in the 1970s. As the name implies, this therapy focuses on relationship conflicts as the source of depression. It tends to be brief – 12 to 16 weeks – and it focuses on one or two problem areas. Specifically, it examines the roles various people play in our lives and our interactions with them. By striving to resolve interpersonal conflicts, it posits that our symptoms and

depression also resolve. Research shows that it is effective as both a standalone treatment for depression and/or in combination with medication.[3]

2. **Psychodynamic Therapy:** This originated from the work of Austrian neurologist Sigmund Freud, MD, PhD, in the late 1800s. This therapy is based on the premise that our current thoughts and feelings, many of which we are unaware of, stem from early childhood experiences and our unconscious mind. This therapy involves the patient freely talking about experiences and identifying patterns of thoughts and feelings, which are then addressed. Insight is the mechanism behind improvement. Psychodynamic therapy typically lasts longer than CBT, DBT, or IPT, as it may last over one year. Recent research has shown that psychodynamic therapy is an effective treatment for depression with long-lasting benefits.[4]

3. **Schema Therapy:** Psychologist and Professor Jeffrey Young, PhD, founded schema therapy. A schema is a pattern of thought or behavior. The basic idea is that many repeat unhelpful or maladaptive schemas – particularly self-defeating thoughts and emotions developed during childhood – through adulthood when our "emotional buttons" are pushed. Schema therapy teaches helpful coping styles in response to such schemas.

Schema therapy is an integrative approach – using CBT, as well as attachment theory (how the parent-child relationship affects our emotional bonds with others), gestalt theory (the whole is greater than the sum of its parts), and psychoanalytic object relations theory (interpersonal relationships from a psychodynamic perspective).

There are 18 maladaptive schemas: abandonment; mistrust or abuse; emotional deprivation; shame; social isolation; dependence or incompetence; vulnerability to harm or illness;

enmeshment or an undeveloped self; failure to achieve; entitlement; lack of self-discipline; subjugation or surrendering to others; self-sacrifice; approval or status-seeking; negativity; emotional inhibition; hypercritical; and punitive. According to the schema model, we engage in schema modes, which are those momentary emotional states and coping styles everyone engages in. The four categories of schema modes are the child mode, the maladaptive coping mode, the maladaptive parent mode, and the healthy adult mode. Additionally, three overlying coping styles to schemas are surrender, avoidance, and overcompensation.[5]

The duration of this therapy is dependent on the condition, but it may go on for a year or longer. Schema therapy is indeed another effective treatment for depression.[6]

How to Seek Therapy

When seeking therapy for depression (or a different mental illness), you will likely seek care through a mental health professional based on word of mouth from healthcare professionals, friends or family, and/or through Internet research. Then you can contact the office, see if they accept your insurance if you have it, and schedule an appointment.

Most therapists use a variety of therapeutic orientations at any given time, usually tailoring their therapies to the particular needs and personality of the client. For example, when dealing with a patient who is experiencing a high degree of interpersonal conflict, that therapist may employ IPT. For a patient with deep-seated past trauma as their central issue, the therapist may employ psychodynamic therapy or refer the client to a therapist who uses that specific therapy.

If you want a particular therapy you have to call and ask, and you may receive services through that counselor or be directed elsewhere. Therapists tend to list conditions they treat, while few advertise their specific therapeutic orientation, although you can try to find a therapist who uses a specific therapy you are seeking. It appears, however, that therapists who offer specific therapies are more apt to be located near big cities, although you might be able to receive counseling from them online.

Examples of agencies to find counselors include the National Association of Cognitive-Behavioral Therapists (NACBT) and the Association for Behavioral or Cognitive Therapies (ABCT). Further, the popular magazine Psychology Today has a search engine to find counselors which may be local to you, or you might be able to seek online counseling through betterhelp.com.

As for your experience with chronic illness, you will inevitably face varying degrees, stages, and time periods of grief and loss when dealing with a chronic illness. How you respond to your chronic illness could mean the difference between adjusting well or succumbing to despair and depression. Fortunately, depression is highly treatable. CBT approaches and the various above therapies – which address thoughts, feelings, and behaviors – offer evidence-based strategies to help you cope more effectively, overcome depression, and live more abundantly.

Chapter 5

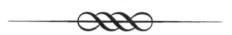

Social Support as a Critical Element

Your relationships profoundly impact the trajectory of your chronic illness. A chronic illness can be extraordinarily isolating. Yet extensive research has revealed that staying socially connected with others and receiving assistance from them in your time of need – known as social support – improves your psychological, cognitive, and physical health, as well as your management of chronic health conditions.[1-2]

More specifically, research shows that social support enhances the functioning of the immune system, endocrine system, and cardiovascular system.[3] Clearly, social support plays a critical role in the management of chronic illness.

Four types of social support are:

1. **Emotional:** showing love and empathy, listening to a problem, and offering encouragement.

2. **Instrumental** (tangible aid or service): walking a dog, cleaning a house, or financial assistance.

3. **Informational:** receiving advice and information from your healthcare professional, a nonprofit organization, or another trustworthy source.

4. **Companionship:** a sense of belonging.

Changes in Friendships During a Chronic Illness

The Greek philosopher Heraclitus once said, "Change is the only constant in life." True in every aspect of life, relationships seem particularly dynamic. Your friendships and the nature of them will change regardless of your health status. As you age, you will make new friends and lose old ones. You will grow closer to certain people and move further away from others. The nature of your long-lasting friendships may change as well, depending on numerous factors such as your family composition, where you live, and your evolving interests. The sooner you can accept and embrace this reality, the better off you will be.

A life-changing event such as a chronic illness presents a unique challenge when it comes to friendships. The challenges may range from needing to cancel or limit social gatherings or outings, concealing your chronic illness from others because of shame and your and/or their uneasiness with your illness (as you may question why others would want to befriend someone so ill), and parting ways with fair-weather friends. A friend of mine with empty nose syndrome (ENS) remarked that sadly "Before ENS, he had many friends. After ENS, they largely disappeared." If your friend falls into the category of "fair-weather," do not sweat it. While painful to lose a friend, you are better off without them.

It is easy to focus on the limitations in friendships imposed by chronic illness, but an invisible chronic illness also presents friendship opportunities – opportunities you would not have if you were in better health. The opportunities include educating existing friends about your illness, making friends through new hobbies or activities, and meeting new friends with a common bond.

I am very fortunate to say that, to some extent, I have enjoyed all of the above. I cherish and value my friendships and I try my best to keep in regular contact with them. Some of my longest friendships, the oldest of which began in 2nd grade, remain strong friendships today and I openly share my medical issues with them. In fact, one of my longstanding friends actively edited my previous book, and he accompanied me to many of my 4 ½ hour trips to my former immunologist. This friend has remained supportive and encouraging through thick and thin.

As I have suffered with chronic illness since 1997, I have also formed many new friendships, particularly at my church, but also through work and other activities. I have also enjoyed forming new friendships with ENS sufferers online. One of my favorite memories was meeting an ENS friend and his wife at the Mayo Clinic in 2008 where we enjoyed a free joint appointment to discuss an ENS research study.

Before commenting further, it is important to note that a chronic illness can make socialization more tiring, and solitude and quietness more refreshing. This is to be expected, and an aspect of chronic illness to which you need to pace yourself and adapt. As an introvert, I admit that I have become more of an introvert as a result of my chronic illness. And that's okay.

Ten Tips for Making and Maintaining Friendships with a Chronic Illness

1. **Actively listen to others.** Talking comes easier for most people than listening. Yet the more you listen to others and remain in touch with them, the closer you will be to them and the more you realize everyone has problems. By listening to your friend's concerns, you will not only build a better understanding of your relationship with them, but hopefully they will also reciprocate and listen to yours.

2. **Openly communicate about your chronic illness.** Determine how much or how little you want to share. Your true

friends will want to be there for you. Sometimes during Bible studies at my church I would withdraw from sharing during discussions, thinking no one could relate. Yet after sharing about my chronic illness, I realized just how sympathetic and understanding some of the leaders have been toward me. And keep in mind: how can we build strong friendships without some level of transparency regarding our chronic illness?

3. **Celebrate your friend's successes.** This may be particularly difficult if you cannot reach the same goal because of your illness. Yet in so doing, you demonstrate an exceptional level of maturity and mental well-being. We naturally tend to look at our situations and assume we have it worse than others. By celebrating others, rather than remaining self-focused and jealous of them, you will likely find yourself happier, appreciated by them, and inspired. You will also know their tips for success, which you can then apply to your own life.

4. **Stay in touch with your friends.** In the hustle and bustle of life, we often lose touch with others. It can be particularly easy to withdraw due to a chronic illness, given its private and burdensome nature and the shame associated with it. You should stay in touch with others to let them know how you are doing, and you may even wish to share whether you are in a flare-up or remission. You could even post updates online as you deem appropriate. Stay in touch on Instagram, Facebook, Snapchat, FaceTime, Skype, and/or through text messaging, emails, or phone calls.

5. **Try to interpret nonverbal cues correctly.** Sizing up a social situation and recognizing if that person wants to be a friend in the first place may be the key when meeting new people. Our body language and tone of voice represent up to 93% of our communication, while the actual words we say represent only

7% of our communication. So watch for the body language of others and monitor your own. Examples of body language include facial expressions, tone of voice, gestures, posture, touch, eye contact, and personal space. For example, is the person you are talking to making good eye contact and nodding, or appearing disinterested with a blank look?

6. **Initiate plans you can keep.** Rather than waiting for others to make plans, do it yourself. By making the plans yourself, you can control the activity and only schedule what you are up for. Perhaps you can plan for a walk in the park or a meal at a restaurant.

7. **Be the friend you want them to be.** Confident friendship-makers assume that others will like them and they do not take rejection personally if they do not. Show you care by smiling, making small talk, complimenting others, and reaching out.

8. **Initiate contact with others.** It is harder work to make friends as adults than as children because children are frequently in a group for long periods with shared experiences, whereas adults have much greater independence, usually much less time together, and more responsibilities. Consequently, adults need to initiate these friendships and reach out to others, especially early in the friendship.

9. **Get in touch with old friends.** Make a phone call to see how your friend is doing. You can also reconnect with your friend through either social media or mutual friends.

10. **Make friendships through online communities.** By joining an online forum with others who have chronic illness, you will likely meet many people who have chronic needs like yours.

One empty nose syndrome Facebook forum, for example, has over 3,000 members.

Dating with a Chronic Illness

The above tips can also be helpful when you are on the dating scene with a chronic illness. For dating, however, I believe you need to be upfront and honest early on. You might in fact wish to share information about your chronic illness *ahead* of your first date (or perhaps shortly thereafter), so that the other person can react privately and process what you shared.

Some might suggest hiding your illness at first to not scare off a potential partner and let true love develop, and that your partner will accept your condition later on; my opinion is this relationship may not end well because the truth will surface and your potential partner may not be ready, willing, or strong enough to handle your chronic illness. After all, strong, successful relationships are built upon open and honest communication. And if that person is scared off and does not show interest in meeting you or continuing the relationship because of your chronic illness, then you can check that person off the list and not waste anyone's time.

Regardless of when and how much (or little) you decide to disclose, just be yourself, have a sense of humor, educate the person about your chronic illness in the right amount of detail, and do not worry about rejection. You are just as worthy of love as anyone else.

Online Support Groups

Active online communities exist for most invisible chronic illnesses, including many rare conditions. What makes them particularly useful is that you can ask questions anonymously and receive responses quickly, often from those with more experience than you. I have found this avenue of support very useful, for example, by posting questions anonymously on the website of the Immune Deficiency Foundation. While online responses cannot replace medical advice, you can learn so much from their responses and then discuss similar thoughts with your healthcare professional. You may also make new friends through these online support groups as you share a common bond in living with chronic illness.

Popular online communities devoted to a variety of illnesses are The Mighty, Healing Well, and the Invisible Disabilities Association. These three online communities include stories, videos, articles, newsletters, and forums where you can connect with others on your chronic illness.

While an online support group can offer wonderful support, it can also become distracting and emotionally draining as you see how much others are suffering. Misery loves company. Additionally, an online support group can be a source of both good and bad information.

You should seek an online community forum with the following:

- ◆ **Active moderators:** They remove spam and address disruptive members and hostile or toxic interactions.

- ◆ **Well-organized topics:** As a result, you know where to post. For example, based upon the organization of the forum, you know where to post about your response to a medication.

- ◆ **Healthcare professionals and/or a medical organization oversee the forum:** This may include reputable physicians on the relevant healthcare topics or a well-established organization.

In-Person and/or Virtual Support Groups

Similar to an online support group, an in-person support group offers another opportunity to fill that gap between a challenging chronic illness and emotional support. This group may be offered through a nonprofit organization, local hospital, or patients. It could also invite an expert for a one-time meeting such as a physician, nurse, or psychologist who could take questions on a topic. It should be noted, however, that an in-person group session does not constitute group counseling or therapy; group psychotherapy involves a licensed mental health professional who counsels a number of people with similar needs. In the event that you cannot find a local in-person group on your condition, meeting face-to-face virtually might be another option, particularly for those with rare conditions.

Whether in-person or virtual, a well-run group should include:

- a facilitator;
- organized topics;
- handouts;
- a place to record contact information.

The benefits of a well-run support group include social connectedness, shared experiences, openly expressing your emotions, exposure to new coping skills and/or treatment strategies, and encouragement. Risks include excessive venting, leaking of confidential information, inappropriate medical advice, and a tendency to compare experiences and conditions.

Mentor

A mentor is an experienced and trusted adviser. Big Brothers Big Sisters, for example, is an organization where older people mentor a younger youth who has experienced adversity. A mentor is someone who has "been there, done that." When I was first diagnosed with an immune deficiency disorder and grappling with this diagnosis, I contacted the Immune Deficiency Foundation who arranged a phone conversation with a mentor. I enjoyed asking this person various questions about living with an immune deficiency disorder as it related to diagnosis, treatment, work, and my life in general. A good mentor should be knowledgeable and patient, show tactfulness when discussing sensitive topics, and demonstrate a stable lifestyle and/or has shown accomplishments despite their illness.

Church

In addition to various community, nonprofit, and government groups from which you can receive social support, church also represents an excellent option. I have a deep faith in Christ and have attended church-related activities all my life. In fact, I got to know my wife, Colleen, through a Bible study we attended together while in college.

My family currently attends a phenomenal and thriving church called Hope Alliance, which is of the Christian and Missionary Alliance denomination, and it offers numerous ministries and opportunities for social support.

On a personal note, the elders pray with me, have anointed me with oil when dealing with sicknesses (as instructed in James 5:13-14), and I have thoroughly enjoyed the instruction and interaction at the men's Bible studies. I feel connected with the members of this church, which has provided me with great social support as I suffer with chronic illness.

Chapter 6

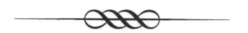

How to Share with Others about your Chronic Illness

Common Misperceptions among Family Members, Friends, and Doctors

Everyone judges everyone. We judge people through both our conscious and unconscious, reflexive thoughts. Our point of view, shaped by numerous prior experiences, drives our understanding of others. Although taught to not judge a book by its cover, we judge all the time, often in a reflexive manner. Upon meeting a new person, we observe that person's appearance, smile, handshake, body language, and mannerisms in the first few seconds (and even *milliseconds*) to make reflexive judgments about his or her trustworthiness and competence.

In addition to this reflexive judgment, we also commit a bias in thinking called the fundamental attribution error (FAE). The FAE asserts that we under-emphasize situation and context reasons to explain behavior while we over-emphasize personal and character traits. We believe the other person's actions reveal who they are. If a chronically ill person states he is not up for going to a store, for example, we may view that person as lazy, rude, complaining, and malingering, even though he is in fact exhausted, in pain, and needs rest.

Interestingly, the reason we commit the FAE is not to understand people better, but to make us feel better about ourselves. So when your chronically ill friend is not up for an outing, the FAE helps you feel better about yourself, as you justify your own actions by thinking, "At least I am acting productive and helpful by going to the store."

We surely apply our reflexive judgments and the FAE toward those with chronic illness. In fact, those with an invisible chronic illness often view chronic illness more empathetically than someone without a chronic illness. This is because they can relate. On the other hand, those without a chronic illness seem more apt to question the diagnosis and the severity of the condition.

Although noted in previous chapters that the person we fight the most emotional battles with is ourselves, misunderstanding and the resulting harsh words from others can also be incredibly painful to the chronically ill. Some will assume, for instance, that a person who is hunched over, uses a walker, or has dementia (an illness with short-term forgetfulness) somehow brought their illness upon themselves and they are inferior, weak, or a lesser human. None of that could be further from the truth. Illnesses happen. In addition, the tough reality is that others often cannot relate or even understand unless they have walked in someone else's shoes.

Not a Valid Diagnosis

Doubting family, friends, co-workers, and even doctors may question your diagnosis and view you as a hypochondriac. This is true for a patient with a diagnosis, and especially before a diagnosis. They think, "Just stop being sick" or "It's all in your head." They solved their occasional acute illnesses, they note, so why cannot you.

Their theories to explain your illness range from:

- Taking medication, the wrong medication, or too much medication.
- Not following a special diet or eating too much dairy.
- Engaging in negative thinking, overthinking, exaggerating, or being preoccupied by it.
- Failing to try acupuncture, herbs, or vitamins.
- Not adhering to a treatment protocol close enough.

♦ Making poor lifestyle choices fully within your control.

When others doubt the validity of your diagnosis, they may accuse you of acting in an attention-seeking or "pity party" manner. They may perceive you as exploiting services, accommodations, or treatments that should be reserved for someone in "greater need." Over time, we may also start to internalize *their* points of view that we are exaggerating our suffering and exploiting services or treatments, which can actually harm us by preventing us from accessing the medications, services, or accommodations we need.

A personal example: some have questioned the validity of my immune deficiency disorder by suggesting that my heavy antibiotic usage caused my chronic infections. While antibiotics do create bacterial resistance and contribute to yeast overgrowth – serious dangers resulting from their overuse – antibiotics do not cause an immune deficiency disorder. Rather, they play an important role in treating infections and immune deficient patients may need to be on them for a longer-than-normal period of time to fully eradicate an infection.

They Question the Severity of your Illness

When others doubt the validity of your illness, they may view you as faking your illness and encourage you to push through it. They struggle to understand why you frequently need to cancel on them, why you are not up for social gatherings or outings, or why you do not appear productive. Although most people with chronic illness would prefer to stay productive than chronically ill any day, they may view you as lazy and over-indulging in rest or your "time off." In short, they often perceive your invisible chronic illness as not severe enough to prevent you from engaging in daily life activities.

Doctors may similarly question the severity of your health condition and accuse you of faking, exaggerating, or over-focusing on your symptoms, or cast doubt on an existing diagnosis or potential diagnosis. This particularly frustrates and disappoints because your honest observation of your symptoms warrant discussion and you need to access healthcare through your doctor. When this happens, remain calm and trust your gut if it is telling you to consider seeking healthcare through a doctor who seems more attuned to your needs; defending yourself can ironically cause abandonment and even self-doubt, particularly if undiagnosed.

They Feel Powerless

When confronted with an invisible chronic illness, many family members, friends, and others feel powerless. They strongly prefer to fix the problem promptly, even though they cannot. They become very uncomfortable when recognizing their helplessness and try to escape this feeling at all costs. Consequently, they may say anything to regain a sense of control over your chronic illness. Through strong feelings and sometimes harsh words they may offer suggestions, criticisms, and even accusations. This can lead to hurt feelings and damaged relationships. In fact, while the average divorce rate is 40%, this jumps to 75% when one spouse has a chronic illness!

When others voice insensitive or even harsh words, remember:

1. **Stay calm.** Cooler heads always prevail. You will never win a power struggle, so do not engage in it.

2. **Think before you speak.** Respond, don't react. You cannot erase what you say, and you could find yourself also saying harsh or hurtful words.

3. **Choose your words wisely.** You want to make sure you convey your precise message, not an unintended one.

4. **It is okay to be quiet in the moment.** You may wish to address this person at later time when all is calm.

5. **Try not to take it personally.** They might misunderstand your illness, not you as a person. Additionally, the person who stated the harsh words might not have meant to hurt you, or even realized how their words affected you.

Nevertheless, when others question the validity of your diagnosis and/or the severity of your symptoms, it can be heartbreaking to have your symptoms and feelings diminished, devalued, mocked, and misjudged. It is discouraging interactions like these, however, that should remind and motivate us to want to educate others about our chronic illness. That said, we have a responsibility to not only educate ourselves about our chronic illness, but also others.

As former President of South Africa (and anti-apartheid activist) Nelson Mandela said: "Education is the most powerful weapon you can use to change the world."

How to Best Inform Others

It can be a balancing act explaining our condition to others. If we conceal our chronic illness from others, we run the risk of them assuming we are in good health. If we stay open and honest about our illness and how it has affected us, others might assume we are over-focusing or complaining about our illness. It takes wisdom to know when and how much to share with others. That said, the following offers guiding thoughts on sharing with others.

We set the tone when educating others about our invisible chronic illness. If we are uneasy about it, others will be too. If we convey how our illness affects us in clear, objective terms, others may seem more at ease about it and understand it better. Of course, how much you decide to share and educate others really depends on a "need-to-know" basis. Only you can decide the correct level of detail to share and only you can gauge if the person you share with seems ready to listen. The closer we are to people, the more we will likely share. After all, if you have a close relationship, you would rather have them hear of your illness directly from you than from another source. This sharing of our experiences with illness, in turn, can improve our relationship with them, as sharing usually leads to increased understanding and support as everyone has their challenges.

When sharing, try to keep it simple, brief, understandable, and familiar; you may wish to avoid sharing gross or technical details. At the same time, communicating on your illness by offering occasional updates with friends or even sharing an occasional status update online, allows you to keep the dialogue open on your chronic illness.

For example, the spoon theory as discussed in chapter 1, offers an explanation for fatigue which is simple, brief, understandable, and familiar. The spoon theory consists of spoons which represent units of energy, limited in supply, and it suggests those with chronic illness use up their spoons surprisingly quickly.

Other considerations for educating others about your invisible chronic illness include:

◆ **Share information from reputable sources.** Examples include an organization's website or peer-reviewed literature with key points highlighted.

◆ **Offer to bring your family member or friend with you to an appointment.** This grants them firsthand insight into your chronic illness.

◆ **Explain your diagnosis and how it has affected your lifestyle in simple, concrete terms.** A back pain sufferer might state, "My chronic lower back pain makes it feel as though I have constant needles in my back while trying to do any task such as taking a shower, walking down the steps, lifting anything, doing any household chores, and sleeping. This lack of sleep, in turn, creates a vicious cycle as my body remains unable to heal from the pain."

♦ **Discuss your illness' long-term prognosis.** If your prognosis is good, you could note that your health condition can remain stable with proper management, but that you may always suffer from some degree of fatigue and pain.

♦ **Explain your treatment plan.** In managing my immune deficiency disorder, I could state, "The immune system produces antibodies to naturally fight infections. Because my body cannot produce enough antibodies on its own, I infuse daily with antibody replacement therapy so I can more effectively fight infections." A second example I could state is "I wash out my sinuses daily because my nose cannot do that on its own and mucus otherwise builds up."

♦ **If your loved one offers misguided advice, acknowledge that you appreciate the support, but *gently* explain why their suggestions are incorrect.** For example, if your loved one suggests following a strict gluten-free diet to cure your rheumatoid arthritis (RA), you might respond, "Thank you for your concern on my health. I believe following an anti-inflammatory diet is important for managing my condition, but a gluten-free diet cannot cure rheumatoid arthritis nor am I convinced that a gluten-free diet can even help rheumatoid arthritis very much because there is only limited evidence of that in the research."

♦ **You may also wish to highlight what you *can* do.** You might note you can still stay productive at your job, volunteer in the community, and/or play a round of tennis.

The previous strategies to inform your loved ones offer no guarantee your loved ones will come to terms with your illness or understand it. In some cases, they may not even *want* to understand it. Losing support from loved ones, especially family, can be very painful and you may need new sources of social support, which you can indeed find as discussed in chapter 5. Nevertheless, the above strategies for educating others represent a strong starting point as they effectively counter the common misperceptions others have about chronic illness.

Inform your Employer (if you must)

Someone with an invisible chronic illness must carefully select what career matches their interests and skills, while staying realistic about their chronic illness. You do not want to pursue a career that will cause you to "push and crash," resulting in endless flare-ups. On the other hand, you do not want to set the bar too low for yourself.

My mother has frequently told me I would have made an excellent doctor, for example, but I know that the gruel of medical school and its impending sense of doom, endless hours of residency, and countless hours in practice as a physician would create endless flare-ups and a vicious downward cycle for my health.

The good news is that there are many careers that can accommodate people with invisible illnesses. It might involve creativity on your part but, with the Internet at your fingertips and an understanding of your strengths and limitations, the possibilities are plentiful. Examples include an online instructor, an online marketer, a graphic designer, and a medical transcriptionist.

Now, after you have carefully selected your career and are employed in it, then you need to determine how much to share with your employer. What you share with your employer should always be determined on a "need-to-know" basis.

Three considerations for how much to disclose to an employer include:

1. If your illness does not interfere with your work responsibilities or your job performance, then you do not need to share anything with your employer. An employer might hear of a progressive health condition and view you as less valuable, which could in turn limit your opportunities for professional advancement. Or if you do feel a need to share with your employer, mention the condition but limit the details.

2. You should determine if you need accommodations before you incur a flare-up, and then seek them. Workplace accommodations include, but are not limited to, working from home, limiting the number of hours or doing flexible hours, a standing desk, a snack on hand, or convenient access to a restroom.

3. The Americans with Disabilities Act (ADA) prohibits discrimination against people with disabilities in all public domains, including school, transportation, and jobs. Keep in mind when applying for an interview with a prospective employer, however, you might decide not to share anything about your chronic illness because, although you receive protections under the ADA, the prospective employer may not hire you and blame the reason on something other than your disability.

The long-term reality of an invisible chronic illness is that flare-ups and remissions will occur, sometimes for extended periods. When you feel your best, you might do a superb job only to find that the following days, weeks, or even months your flare-up continuously interferes with your job performance. In that case, you should have a plan B for employment – a worst case scenario. This can be stressful, particularly as you rely on your employment for health insurance and survival.

During the coronavirus pandemic, many people in office jobs worked from home to prevent the spread of the coronavirus. For example, although just a temporary arrangement, I attended many virtual Committee on Special Education meetings, wrote reports, made phone calls, and attended virtual conferences. Likewise, telecommuting offers an alternate career in which you can work from home.

In the event, however, your illness impacts your ability to perform a job at all and you live in the United States, then you may need to apply for disability through the United States Social Security administration so you can receive government assistance to cover your living expenses. In order to receive disability, there is a five month waiting period from the point when you first became disabled. Furthermore, your disability should render you unable to engage in any "substantial gainful activity" and your disability should be expected to continue for at least another year.

Educate the Politicians and Exercise your Right to Vote

In September 2019, due to her passing, I became aware of Marca Bristo who had once attended the school where I am a practicing school psychologist. Marca Bristo, a strong advocate for people with disabilities, broke her neck when diving into shallow water in Lake Michigan in 1977. As a result of this accident, she was paralyzed from the chest down. In addition to losing her job, income, and health insurance, she quickly realized that people with disabilities faced inaccessibility to bathrooms, buses, various public and private facilities, and even restaurants.

Rather than dwell on her loss, she focused on what she could do – and did she ever! She played a key role in drafting the Americans with Disabilities Act of 1990 (ADA). She chaired the American National Council on Disability from 1994 to 2002, she served as president of the United States International Council on Disabilities in 2014, and she was also president of Access Living Metropolitan Chicago. Through her political advocacy, she educated the politicians and made a groundbreaking difference in the lives of the disabled.

You, too, can make a difference in the lives of those with invisible chronic illnesses through education and advocacy. You might think your efforts do not matter or seem insignificant, but as Marca Bristo demonstrated, your efforts do matter and you can make a difference.

You can:

- ◆ Volunteer with an organization devoted to your health condition.

- ◆ Contact political leaders regarding legislation and/or matters relevant to your health.

- ◆ Use your talents through various social media platforms (e.g., writing, doing graphic design, or fundraising).

You can also make a difference by voting. However, it can be difficult to get out and vote when you have an invisible chronic illness. In July 2020, USA Today wrote an article entitled *30 years after the ADA, access to voting for people with disabilities is still an issue.*[1] The article cited parking spaces, ramps, wheelchair inaccessibility, nonworking voting machines, and even mail-in ballots that do not accommodate the blind, as barriers for voting.

Yet voting offers the most direct path to influence change for people with disabilities. If you contact your elected official, they will first check if you are registered to vote, and they will be far more inclined to act on your request if you are a registered voter. So it is imperative you exercise your right to vote.

Various pieces of legislation passed throughout the years have made a tremendous difference for those with invisible chronic illnesses, including the Social Security Act §223, the Americans with Disabilities Act of 1990 (ADA), and the Family and Medical Leave Act (FMLA).

In recent years, proposed legislation included an item to move disability reviews, which are mostly completed on invisible illnesses, from every 3 years to every 2 years. The goal of this move is to save money by removing people from benefits. Thankfully, this change was denied based upon the votes of the people. Your role as a voter, and the difference it can make in the lives of those with invisible chronic illnesses, cannot be overstated.

Advocate for your Illness

It is inspiring to imagine what one person or a small group of people can do when they put their minds to it. Consider Wayne and Sherri Connell. Authors of *But You LOOK Good, How to Encourage and Understand People Living with Illness and Pain,* Wayne and Sherri founded the Invisible Disabilities Association in 1996. In part due to the level of misunderstanding Sherri incurred as a sufferer with multiple sclerosis and Lyme disease, this organization started with the mission of properly defining and raising awareness on invisible disabilities. The Invisible Disabilities Association has grown tremendously and has done an incredible job of their stated mission of encouraging, educating, and connecting people with invisible disabilities throughout the world.

Stories like this should encourage us to do our part as well. We may not be able to lead millions worldwide, but educating others on a social media forum, sharing your story with a loved one, or creating useful videos are all valuable forms of advocacy.

Chapter 7

How Loved Ones Can Support You

An invisible chronic illness creates not only undue stress and challenges for you, but also on your loved ones, including your coworkers, friends, family, and particularly your spouse – who in some cases is your caregiver. The following tips and suggestions can equip your loved one so they can best support you in your journey with chronic illness, as well as take care of themselves. This chapter is written directly to and for them. It is broken down into what they should and should not say, what they can do, as well as how a well spouse (who may also be a caregiver) can support you and themselves.

So, if you are a coworker, friend, family member, spouse, caregiver, or someone who knows someone with a chronic illness, your words and actions can have a tremendous impact on their suffering, for better or worse. You may want to help your family member or friend, but aren't sure what to say or do, or what they really need. This chapter will show you exactly how you can help your chronically ill loved one.

What you Can Say

In addition to listening to your friend or loved one with a chronic illness, which can do wonders in and of itself, what you say to your loved one can make or break his or her day. A 10-minute encounter and the words you say can have a potent impact on their mood for the remainder of their day, few days, weeks, or longer. So choose your words wisely, but do not worry too much if you do not have all the right words in the moment. The actual words you say make up only a small part of your communication, while your nonverbal communication makes up the rest. Plus, your heart behind your words makes the larger difference.

Your supportive words toward your loved ones generally fall into one of the following three categories:

1. Your words validate their illness and feelings.

2. Your words indicate your caring interest in them as a person and their illness.

3. Your words demonstrate flexibility, understanding, and that you are not judgmental.

Below are 10 different statements – which fall into the above three categories – that you can say to your loved one with a chronic illness:

1. **"I believe you."** And do genuinely believe them. Chronic illness patients commonly feel misunderstood. They encounter people who do not believe them, downplay their illness, or judge them. These three simple words offer perhaps the most powerful statement you can make. The chronically ill generally don't seek sympathy, but understanding. Saying "I believe you" validates their illness and comforts them, and it offers a deeper connection with the chronically ill than almost any other statement.

2. **"That is horrible."** Another example of validating your loved one's suffering, these words convey the seriousness and impact of their illness. You are not attempting to "fix" their illness, but keeping it simple and focused on them. Of course, if your loved one does not view her illness as "horrible," she will clarify and elaborate on how she does view her illness. Your loved one will also be more inclined to open up about her chronic illness without feeling like she is complaining or her feelings are being diminished and devalued.

3. **"It must be devastating to be so sick all the time."** This statement shows not only that you listened to your loved one, but also that you validate his or her concerns. Instead of "devastating," you could also use terms such as "exhausting," "grueling," "horrible," or "very difficult," depending on the situation. Your loved one will appreciate your validation no matter which words you choose.

4. **"You look good, but how are you really feeling?"** A similar remark you could make is "Tell me what is going on." Or a third way to inquire is "Do you believe you have made progress since your initial diagnosis?" Those with an invisible chronic illness usually do not look sick, which contributes to the misunderstanding. These statements show your interest in them and their chronic illness. You cannot read their minds, *which may be a good thing*, but they may be reluctant to share otherwise as they do not want to come across as complaining. By showing you care and want to understand, it offers them an opportunity to openly share their symptoms and progress.

5. **"You should be proud of yourself for how hard you're trying."** You could also say "You seem so strong for what you have endured." Your loved one often has to work much, much harder than others to achieve similar goals. Living with a chronic illness that requires continual management and results in frequent flare-ups can be challenging, to put it mildly.

Chronic illness often leads to shame and self-blame, as your loved one's chronic illness serves as a constant reminder of his limitations. He often feels guilty for not doing more, with a tendency to overdo it. Stating the importance of pride in oneself shows not only validation of his illness, but also reminds him of his hard work and successes along the way.

6. **"Your illness is not your fault."** Not merely validating their illness, this is a simple reminder to refrain from self-blaming. It further shows your loved one that you do not blame her for her illness, but in fact, are trying to understand it and recognize that she is doing her best.

7. **"I hope you are as well as possible."** Your loved one with a chronic illness may not get well. When talking with others about chronic illness – unless if they face an acute crisis such as an infection which they can fully heal from – I try to refrain from saying "Get well" or "I hope you feel better." In so doing, I recognize that the chronically ill remain unable to completely heal from their illness. Stating "as well as possible" validates this reality, and removes the pressure from your loved one to feel better if they cannot, but acknowledges you want their health to improve from its current state.

8. **"I am not sure what to say, but I am here for you."** Your presence matters. Finding the right words can be challenging for anyone, but particularly if you do not fully understand or cannot personally relate to your loved one's illness. That's okay. Your actions speak louder than words. Chronic illness can be very lonely and isolating. Staying present with them shows you care about them and offers a great amount of comfort in and of itself.

9. **"I understand if you need to cancel plans at the last minute."** Or if he is running behind, you could state "I understand if you are running behind." These statements show your flexibility in response to your loved one's chronic illness. It also takes the pressure and guilt off your loved one from feeling like he must not cancel or be running late no matter how lousy he feels or what he needs to do.

10. **"I am going to Walmart. Can I pick up anything for you?"**
This statement is specific and is likely to be acted upon, unlike the statement, "If you need anything, let me know." A similar statement could be, "I would like to come over to your home today. Is there anything I could bring you?" Your loved one may really need help, but she does not wish to feel like a burden on you. Both statements show your willingness to bring her something and your flexibility in adapting to her needs. Or, instead of asking, you could simply pick up a treat you know she enjoys to make her day a little brighter.

While it is important to address your loved one's chronic illness, please note he or she might also want a break from discussing the pain or illness. We all need breaks and there is so much more to life than chronic illness. So you might want to talk about other topics as well and give space if it is needed.

What you should Not Say

While supportive words are encouraging, careless, insensitive, and especially well-intentioned but misguided words can deflate your loved one with chronic illness – much more than you realize. The words you use can either lift them up or tear them down. While these words are difficult to hear from a coworker or friend, they tend to be particularly hurtful if you are a family member, spouse, or caregiver of someone with a chronic illness. Unsupportive words send the message that either you doubt or minimize their illness, that you view their illness as solely mental in nature, that you judge them, and/or that you do not understand their chronic illness.

Below are 10 common statements that you should not say to someone with a chronic illness:

1. **"You don't look sick."** This is similar to "You look fine." Most people with a chronic illness do not look sick, which is why I

titled this book, *Finding Joy with an Invisible Chronic Illness.* This statement subtly implies you do not believe they are as sick as they report. Yet how they look typically has nothing to do with how they feel or what they experience on a daily basis.

2. **"You cannot be that sick if you have worked or volunteered for __ number of years."** While you openly doubt the severity of their sickness, the fact they have worked or volunteered for some number of years might just mean that your loved one with chronic illness is a *warrior.*

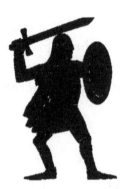

3. **"It's all in your head."** This one is about as bad as the "stay positive" advice so often given to chronic illness sufferers. When doctors do not understand a physical illness, they frequently chalk it up to psychological origins. This comment similarly stems from ignorance. Your loved one has a real physical illness and positive thinking will not cure it. Positive thinking offers a valuable tool in their journey, but the chronically ill should not deny or avoid the negative emotions that a chronic illness can elicit. Rather, they need to confront the negative emotions, thinking patterns, and physical challenges associated with an invisible chronic illness so they can move forward in managing it.

4. **"Have you ever tried___?"** The answer is yes. You name it and your chronic illness warrior has tried it! And they likely have done an amazing job at trying countless unhelpful remedies. Suggesting that your loved one should try a certain diet or an expensive supplement or an exercise routine to become "cured" from their chronic illness is not only unhelpful if not insulting, but it also invalidates their illness. Yet regrettably, this offering of limited evidence remedies happens all the time.

5. **"Everyone gets tired or has issues."** While true, your everyday issues and problems are typically much smaller and easier to deal with than a debilitating chronic illness. For example, many chronic illness patients deal with relentless, debilitating fatigue. By minimizing their suffering and brushing off their symptoms, you make an unfair comparison and invalidate their illness.

6. **"It could be worse."** A similar statement is "At least it's not cancer." *Never* compare illnesses. No one wins when you do that. Usually, worse conditions do exist, but by comparing one chronic illness to another, you minimize the seriousness of your loved one's chronic illness. Each chronic illness is unique and can be devastating in its own right.

7. **"I know how you feel."** Chronic illness is a life-changing event that requires continual management and frequent flare-ups and remissions. Even among patients with the same chronic illness, experiences and symptoms can differ drastically. Saying "I cannot imagine how you must feel," on the other hand, offers a much more validating and understanding statement, and it allows your chronically ill loved one to want to explain their illness. Many with an invisible chronic illness would opt to have a more recognized and visible illness – even if more severe – to simply avoid the frequent misunderstandings from others.

8. **"Just push through it or don't focus on it so much."** Like the "no pain, no gain" mentality, this message tells your loved one to work harder and puts unnecessary pressure on them, while implying their symptoms will self-correct with time. Your loved one may already push themselves to their max. Examples include that they might socialize longer than they should, stay longer at a musical event than they should, work harder at their jobs than their body can handle, all in an attempt to fit in and "push through." With chronic illness, pushing yourself to an extent is helpful, but without the proper pacing, pushing too much can be harmful, like taking one step forward but five steps back.

9. **"You must like the attention you get from doctors and your time resting at home."** Most chronically ill patients would prefer to stay far away from doctor's offices if they could. They would also rather stay very productive at work and enjoy a more active and potentially fulfilling life than bedridden and dealing with continual symptoms at home any day. These insulting statements suggest that you do not believe they need the help they receive from healthcare professionals, or the rest they need at home.

10. **"I wish you would stop canceling on me."** Your loved one with a chronic illness wants to stay connected with you, but may feel alone and even guilty about cancelling. They may just not be physically up for an outing.

What you Can Do

Your actions speak louder than words. Your actions, no matter how small, can make a big, positive difference in the life of your loved one with a chronic illness.

When considering how to help, however, don't overdo it. Well-meaning and empathetic family and friends can inadvertently disempower the chronically ill by doing too much for them. The trick is balancing your assistance in a helpful way. One way of doing that is to discuss with the chronically ill individual what he or she can and cannot do. Finding important tasks for the person to do is, in fact, extremely beneficial in helping them feel like they are a contributing member of the family or community.

Furthermore, some of what you perceive as helpful to your loved one may not be helpful at all. Examples of unhelpful actions include visiting an exhausted friend, offering food with nuts despite their food allergy to nuts, or offering a get well card as your loved one cannot get well.

On the other hand, your loved one will likely appreciate that which shows you think and care about them, offers practical help, and provides an opportunity for them to enjoy life more fully or distract them from their illness.

Below are various practical actions and gifts your chronically ill loved one may appreciate, although it may be a good idea to ask what they would like the most before acting on any of them:

1. **Shop for your loved one.** Tell your loved one you are going to the store and ask if you can pick up anything for them or offer to pick up a treat.

2. **Help your loved one with household chores.** Because women tend to complete a majority of household chores in most families, although men living alone would also benefit from this help, this suggestion tends to apply more if your chronically ill loved one is female. Examples include cleaning the kitchen and bathroom, vacuuming the carpet, and doing the laundry.

3. **Offer to take your loved one for a drive, for a trip, and/or for a walk.**

4. **Bring your loved one to the zoo, sporting event, concert, or play.**

5. **Deliver a meal to your loved one or take your loved one to a restaurant or a place they enjoy.**

6. **Offer a hug as you see appropriate.** My wife's grandmother had a reputation for giving hugs to others, and my family and I were of course some of the fortunate recipients. These hugs expressed her love for us. You can do the same.

7. **You could send your loved one a card, flowers, or chocolates to let them know you are thinking of them.**

8. **Buy your loved one a book.** Select an interesting, inspirational, or humorous book, depending on what they enjoy reading.

9. **Give your loved one a gift card to a restaurant or to a place they enjoy.**

10. **Buy your loved one a movie or a series of a favorite show.**

The bottom line is you can do any or all of the above, which show you care. But bear in mind that simply staying present with your loved one can also make a tremendous difference. Listening to them and showing your love, support, and understanding can make a world of difference.

When you are the Well Spouse and/or Caregiver

While *Finding Joy* focuses on the chronically ill, your needs as the well spouse and/or caregiver also merit attention. As the well spouse and particularly if you are also the caregiver, your needs cannot be overstated. One study showed that caregiving partners of someone with a chronic illness reported a lower quality of life than the chronically ill patient him or herself![1]

The dual role of spouse and caregiver can be particularly demanding and labor-intensive. This role may result in feeling overwhelmed and underappreciated, often at the expense of your own needs. Consequently, this dual role results in high levels of depression and burnout – exhaustion, stress, sleep disturbance, loss of interest and sad thoughts, resulting in an attitude shifting from positive and caring to detached and unconcerned.

To exacerbate the situation, your chronically ill loved one may remain polite and upbeat with acquaintances and the outside world, but he or she will likely unleash the brunt of their emotions at home. My colleague refers to this phenomenon as "house devil, street angel."

On top of that, it can be difficult to see your loved one suffer and, at times, to gauge the level of their suffering because they always seem to be sick. So, if you are the well spouse and/or caregiver, you have needs, too.

Providing spousal caregiver support can be demanding and expensive, particularly for the middle class. In many instances, the affluent can afford to hire caregivers out of pocket, while the low income receive Medicaid waivers for hiring caregiver support. One middle income family with a wife who had an invisible chronic illness, for example, received $4,900 per month in take home pay in 2019, and paid out $15,648 that year in home health care, which amounted to a little over $1,300 per month.[e] As a result of these high out-of-pocket costs for caregiving support for the middle class, the spouse often becomes the main caregiver.

According to research published in the International Journal of Epidemiology, men are more likely to develop chronic illness in their lives than women due to modifiable lifestyle habits.[2] Consequently, more women than men tend to play the role of spousal caregiver, and they tend to be more comfortable in this role than men, such as with doing personal care tasks. However, an increasing number of men also find themselves in the role of spousal caregiver, which can be particularly taxing on a family as women historically tend to do the bulk of caregiving, including household chores, meals, and child-rearing.

Regardless of your gender, however, you and your chronically ill spouse need to develop a plan for addressing the major issues in life.

Below are seven topics on which you and your ill spouse should jointly discuss and determine:

1. **Finances for healthcare.** Money matters cause marital conflict more than any other issue, and managing a chronic illness is expensive. You and your spouse need to figure out your mindset in budgeting for healthcare needs. Does your mindset align with "healthcare at any cost" because you believe you cannot put a price tag on health, or "healthcare within a budget" which recognizes the need for some spending on healthcare, but tries to contain healthcare spending as much as possible? In pursuing healthcare, you may also weigh financing options, hospital discounts, or the expenses of specific healthcare services, which can vary considerably depending on where and to whom you go.

---

[e] The cost of hiring a home health aide for this family was a minimum of $1,600 per month, which covers 20 hours per week, and this does not include household chores, just strictly medical care.

2. **Breaks.** You need them. The role of spousal caregiver can be exhausting, and you need to take care of yourself and enjoy breaks from this role. Hopefully you can talk with your spouse about getting a break at times, even if that means doing an activity your spouse is unable to do. Even an hour break per day or per week can be refreshing.

3. **Chores.** Prior to your spouse's chronic illness, a balance of household and yard chores likely existed in which one spouse completes certain chores while the other does other ones. Every family is different in how these chores are distributed between spouses. Due to chronic illness, these chores may need to be done differently so that both partners share a similar load, in accordance with what they are able to do. For example, men, if your wife has the chronic illness, you may need to do more household cleaning, cook more, or plan meals in advance. Or women, if your husband has the chronic illness, you may need to help unclog the sink, go up on a ladder to change the lightbulb, or mow the lawn.

4. **Therapy.** In caring for your spouse, your loss and subsequent grieving is legitimate, too. As noted, your quality of life might suffer more than your spouse's. Plus, you may feel sad for what happened to your partner and need to go through the grieving process. Or you may deal with some level of anger, anxiety, and depression. In either case, you may wish to seek individual or family therapy to help you cope.

5. **Home setting.** You might wish to consider downsizing or decluttering to simplify your life.

6. **Socialization.** You may need to set limits on socialization with others depending on your spouse's health. This may mean

limiting the amount of time you spend with – or how often you get together with – a family friend.

7. **Extended family.** In dealing with your extended family, you should take the lead in educating them about your spouse's physical health needs. You may need to limit visits, and your spouse should also see how they can play a role in this matter. For example, if cake triggers a flare-up for your spouse, then he or she could just politely decline cake at the family gathering.

Lastly, as the spouse and/or caregiver, your needs clearly matter as well. Just like with chronic illness, this role can be lonely. The Well Spouse Association is an organization that offers support for the well spouse. This organization offers a wealth of information and resources, including a forum on which you can connect with others in your situation.

Ultimately, do your best to encourage your loved one with the words you say and the actions you take, but also make sure to take care of yourself. If your needs go unaddressed and you experience burnout in assisting your spouse, then everyone will be affected and will eventually lose out. Your needs matter, too.

Chapter 8

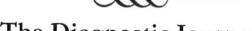

The Diagnostic Journey

The Critical First Steps

R ecognize a problem exists. Then seek to deeply understand it. Take these critical first steps in your diagnostic journey. You may have suffered with various symptoms your entire life, or your symptoms – relentless fatigue, enduring aches and pains, constantly unrefreshing sleep, or unusual or difficult-to-treat infections – began in your adulthood. In either case, solving any medical problem requires awareness that a problem exists, persistence to identify the diagnosis, and a complete understanding of it. You really should not pursue treatments, particularly expensive treatments, if you do not hold at least a basic understanding of your chronic illness.

Granted, many invisible chronic illnesses take an enormous amount of time to understand and learn – for patients and medical professionals alike – and I will be the first to admit I am still learning about mine. The amount of new research on various chronic ailments and their treatments constantly increases, sometimes exponentially, and what is best practice today for treating a chronic illness may change tomorrow. The Internet rapidly accelerates this learning curve.

But that should not discourage you from seeking a strong understanding of your specific illness. You really, really need a clear understanding of your chronic illness. A clear understanding will save you an incredible amount of time, energy, frustration, and expense.

Self-educating Vs. Self-diagnosing

Before going any further, I need to clarify the patient's role between self-educating and self-diagnosing. Chronically ill patients should self-educate, but not self-diagnose. Self-educating facilitates understanding of our illnesses and our bodies, our understanding of the prognosis (the course of an illness), and it can enhance the collaboration between us and our doctors, so it can be tremendously beneficial. I enjoy reading consensus articles on UpToDate, browsing the latest research through PubMed, and even occasionally reading medical journal articles. Perusing and/or participating on Internet forums on different health conditions also increases our learning curve, as we share our experiences and learn from others.

Yet we absolutely need to respect the extensive medical training and knowledge of our healthcare professionals. Unless if our diagnosis is firmly established, we should refrain from undoubtedly asserting we have this condition or that condition, so therefore we need this medication or that MRI. Not only may you be incorrect on the diagnosis, but expect to face great resistance from your healthcare provider who might otherwise be very eager to collaborate with you to pinpoint your condition and find reasonable solutions.

Self-educating Vs. An Official Diagnosis

Granted, the Internet offers a vast powerhouse of information and has helped tremendously with getting the word out on obscure, complex, and rare diseases. For example, I accredit the Internet as being more beneficial for raising awareness on empty nose syndrome (ENS) among the general public than any other factor. I am extremely grateful for the Internet. Our understanding of complex and chronic diseases has increased exponentially because of the Internet.

But with this vast amount of information comes the vast potential to confuse and misdiagnose, particularly with a frightening sounding diagnosis you likely do not have, which will lead to unnecessary anxiety.

The Internet has a vast array of false information, it does not know you, and it cannot offer necessary context. Your persistent cough and hoarseness, for instance, may in fact be a symptom of bronchitis, not cancer. Your chest pain may be a direct result of muscle strain, not an impending heart attack. On the other hand, your much less troubling, but no less nagging symptom of unexplained fatigue may indicate chronic fatigue syndrome, or worse yet, cancer. Absolutely investigate your symptom, collect information, and share pertinent details with your healthcare professional, but leave the official diagnosis to your medical provider. After all, no amount of Internet research can replace the skills of an experienced provider.

That said, most patients with a chronic illness will naturally research their symptoms and self-diagnose, which can feel validating and useful as you seek to understand your condition. In fact, most will overanalyze, myself included. After all, healthcare professionals may not properly or promptly diagnose complex conditions, they are pressed for time, they may diagnose incorrectly, and you want answers to your health ailment. You know you have symptoms and you need an explanation for them. And even without an official diagnosis, you still need just as much help as someone with a diagnosis. In these circumstances, having an improved understanding of your condition through self-educating can be useful and offer some degree of relief in your journey toward an official diagnosis.

Despite the practical value of self-educating, the importance of obtaining an official diagnosis from a healthcare professional cannot be overstated. An official diagnosis offers irrefutable proof of your condition. Additionally, you will find it an uphill battle to access adequate medical care from a healthcare professional without an official diagnosis. I can speak firsthand in that I found obtaining adequate antibiotic management from a medical provider without an official diagnosis of an immune deficiency disorder stressful, to put it mildly, while being treated by a knowledgeable immunologist with an official diagnosis in hand eliminated most of the stress.

Yet it may take time to receive the correct diagnosis, and it is important we are patient with our healthcare professionals if we do not receive a diagnosis right away. Despite a medical system in which the diagnosis guides treatment and the insurance company reimburses based upon diagnostic codes – and although early diagnosis is important so we can intervene and take preventative measures – a fast diagnosis is not *always* in our best interest. We may simply have to observe symptoms for a period of time as some will resolve, others will persist, and still others will change and/or worsen. In these cases, the diagnosis will become clearer over time and you want to be treating the correct illness, not an incorrect one based on a rushed and faulty diagnosis.

Lastly, while an official diagnosis represents a huge step forward in the management of your condition, it also represents a new beginning in your journey of further seeking help for your condition, not the end. In dealing with a chronic illness, the search for improved health and a better quality of life never ceases. Likewise, despite an official diagnosis, you will continue to confront challenges when accessing quality healthcare or dealing with others, but it will be that much easier to confront these challenges. You have cleared a major hurdle.

Beyond the Diagnosis

A diagnosis is not the endpoint when seeking understanding of your condition. Other factors important to understand about your illness include the onset of symptoms and the prognosis.

The onset of symptoms differs among illnesses. A condition such as multiple sclerosis may show few symptoms early on, but result in organ damage during its latter years. Other conditions such as chronic fatigue syndrome include symptoms that surface right away and seem to persist.

Additionally, some illnesses get worse over time while others remain remarkably stable. The prognosis differs based upon the specific illness. The prognosis for some immune deficiency disorders is good with proper treatment, while other conditions – such as multiple sclerosis, Parkinson's disease, and bronchiectasis – worsen over time. Even though they tend to worsen over time, however, not all necessarily will. For example, treatment with immune globulin can slow down the progression of bronchiectasis, and some patients report stable bronchiectasis over many years. For these reasons, diagnostic certainty tends to be clearer than its prognosis, as it can be difficult to predict the future progression of an illness.

A Team Process

As a school psychologist, part of my role is conducting thorough assessments to determine a child's skill level and what educational and related services he or she may need. For each assessment, I share and discuss my findings with other professionals on a multi-disciplinary team. This assessment involves consulting with other professionals; conducting classroom observations; completing interviews with the parents, teachers, and the student; reviewing available, pertinent educational records, including progress monitoring data; and lastly, testing specifically tailored to the area in question. Needless to say, it takes a lot of time to investigate and, only after extensive investigation has been done, can I make appropriate and practical recommendations. And even then, my recommendations may be rightfully challenged by someone who knows the child much better than me. As a result, the Committee on Special Education will consider my expertise, the teacher's expertise, parental insights, and other specialists' vantage points when making any decision on the disability designation and on what type of services the child needs.

In the same way, diagnosing a chronic illness may look a bit like that, a team process – with you, your primary care provider, your medical specialists, perhaps your mental health professionals, and sometimes your friend or family member – making up the team.

Primary Care Provider

Your primary care provider (PCP) should be at the center of your healthcare team, and you will likely present your symptoms first to your PCP before going to specialists. If you live in the United States or a different country and have health insurance, for instance, you should select an in-network PCP, meaning they participate with your insurance, so that you can receive the discounted rates that your insurance company has pre-arranged with your provider. Your PCP may have training in pediatrics (with children), geriatrics (with the elderly), obstetricians/gynecologists (OB/GYN) (with women), internal medicine (adults), or family or general practice (all ages). The following practice as PCPs: a doctor of medicine (MD), which is a traditionally-trained physician; an OB/GYN (for women); and a doctor of osteopathic medicine (DO), which is a holistic-oriented physician with training in musculoskeletal/osteopathic techniques. Nurse practitioners and physician assistants also practice as PCPs, but usually under the supervision of a licensed physician.

As a chronically ill patient, you should select your PCP wisely. In addition to managing common health conditions, your PCP should act as your "medical home base" as he or she coordinates your care with your specialists. You should feel comfortable and confident in your provider. Your PCP must be on board with *all of your diagnoses*, as he or she will be coordinating your care across specialties and making referrals. In collaboration with your PCP, you will be making important decisions about treatment options, such as discussing the risks and benefits of specific treatments versus the risks and benefits of doing nothing. Additionally, your PCP will likely be filling out any paperwork for short or long-term care, disability, or medical leave should you need it.

Furthermore, you will likely need to discuss personal topics with your PCP so you should feel comfortable doing that.

While online reviews and information along with word of mouth provide valuable information, online information may not be up-to-date. A doctor may be listed as "accepting new patients," for instance, when he or she is not and possibly has even left the practice. Further, online reviews may be more reflective of disgruntled patients than representative of how the doctor's patients actually feel, so they should be interpreted with a grain of salt.

You will likely save time by either calling up and inquiring with the healthcare system's main phone line of a potential PCP or, better yet, by calling a potential PCP's office and asking to speak with the office manager. If the PCP is taking new patients, you could then state your diagnosis and/or primary symptoms and, if the PCP has managed other patients with similar needs, talk about what is most important to you in your search for a PCP and thereby determine if the doctor might be a good match. Teaching hospitals offer great options when selecting a PCP because of their longer appointment times, deeper expertise, and close contact with specialists.

Other factors to consider when selecting a PCP: location; convenient office hours; whether you are more comfortable discussing personal issues with a male or female doctor or with a doctor of a certain cultural background; convenience in scheduling an appointment; friendliness of staff; and background and expertise of the PCP.

If, for whatever reason, you cannot find a suitable PCP, then you may wish to include a family member or friend who can help you with coordinating your care across specialists and accompanying you to doctor appointments; in fact, it is almost always beneficial to have a family member or friend accompany you to appointments. When not having a flare-up, not having a PCP may be feasible, but when you are exhausted and too sick to communicate well, this communication can quickly become difficult and your family member or friend is worth their weight in gold.

Medical Specialists

Your PCP will likely refer you to a specialist who can help manage your care, although you can also self-refer to a specialist if you have insurance which allows it. In addition to your PCP's recommendation, for example, other ways to select a specialist include recommendation of advocacy groups, state level associations, online reviews (e.g., Healthgrades, Vitals, and Yelp), family members, friends, colleagues, or healthcare professionals.

Most specialists help in the management of chronic illness. The specialist offers a larger, more tailored toolkit than the PCP for specific illnesses.

In some cases, a physician with a specialty in one area (e.g., pulmonology), may primarily treat patients using their particular expertise in a different area of medicine (e.g., sleep medicine). Similarly, many chronically ill patients have multiple conditions and see multiple specialists, and many specialists are board-certified in more than one area.

Specialists involved in the management of chronic illness include:

- ◆ **Endocrinologist:** a physician trained in hormone disorders who treats conditions such as thyroid disorders, adrenal disorders, and diabetes.

- ◆ **Rheumatologist:** a physician trained in rheumatics – joints, tendons, ligaments, muscles, and bones – who treats inflammatory, autoimmune conditions such as osteoarthritis, rheumatoid arthritis, lupus, and Ehlers-Danlos syndrome (EDS).

◆ **Pain medicine specialists:** a physician trained in pain who treats chronic pain conditions such as complex regional pain syndrome (CRPS), sciatica, and/or other back or neck pain.

◆ **Pulmonologist:** a physician trained in lung disorders who treats conditions such as COPD, cystic fibrosis, and asthma.

Mental Health Professionals

In addition to receiving medical care, you may also require mental health support. The mental health professionals below offer a variety of overlapping services, but there are key differences among them.

Four examples of mental health providers and their key differences include:

◆ **Psychiatrist:** a physician who prescribes medication, diagnoses mental health and medical conditions and can offer psychotherapy, although more commonly does not provide psychotherapy.

◆ **Psychologist:** typically holds a doctoral degree although some psychologists, such as school psychologists and industrial-organizational psychologists, hold at least a master's degree. A licensed psychologist provides therapy and can comprehensively assess and diagnose mental health conditions, but generally cannot prescribe medication. As of this writing, however, licensed psychologists may prescribe in the following 5 states: Iowa, Idaho, Illinois, New Mexico, and Louisiana, as well as in the Public Health Service, the Indian Health Service, the U.S. military, and Guam.

◆ **Social worker:** typically holds at least a master's degree, and can both diagnose and provide therapy for patients with mental health disorders. They focus on connecting patients with community resources.

♦ **Counselor:** typically holds at least a master's degree, and can diagnose and provide therapy for patients with mental health disorders. They focus on providing guidance to patients through therapy sessions.

How to Advocate for Your Needs

When self-advocating for your needs, you should not only choose your team wisely, but also ensure your team communicates well with each other so that they are advocating *for* you and not *against* you. Further, you should continually monitor your health and its progress, or lack thereof, over time.

You might ask yourself the following questions:

♦ Are your symptoms improving, staying the same, or getting worse?

♦ Are you taking the correct medicines?

♦ Are your questions being answered?

♦ Is your doctor listening to your concerns?

♦ Is your doctor accessible?

♦ Are you getting your test results in a timely manner?

♦ Is your doctor providing good insights and suggestions?

Based on the answers to the above questions, you could either stay with your present doctor or be willing to make a change to a different one.

Clearly, awareness that your problem exists and a deep understanding of your medical condition serve as vital precursors to accessing high quality medical care. An official diagnosis, although a critical step forward in the management of your condition, represents the beginning of your health journey, not the end, in your ceaseless pursuit of better health. Further, it is important to bear in mind that illnesses differ with respect to symptom onset and prognosis.

Ultimately, through a strong understanding of your healthcare condition via extensive self-education and if possible, an official diagnosis, and a carefully selected healthcare team to which you continually monitor, you will find it much easier to access the high quality healthcare you need and deserve.

Chapter 9

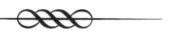

Access and Maintain Quality Healthcare

Before Your Appointment

It can be intimidating and stressful going to a healthcare professional. Most physicians are often pressed for time, with an average office visit time for a specialist ranging from 13 to 24 minutes.[2] These doctors and their assistants often follow a prescribed routine. For example, after the nurse checks your vital signs, updates your medication list, and discusses the reason for your office visit, the doctor enters the room and discusses test results or presenting concerns, and does or recommends specific tests, if indicated. That is why you need to plan for your appointment – to maximize your time and outcome from your appointment. Your plan will also reduce any anxiety you may have. You need to be prepared and concise, knowing the purpose *before* you go.

The more details your healthcare professional knows, the more he or she will be able to accurately diagnose your problem and develop an effective treatment plan. What you can do during your journey of seeking a diagnosis and self-educating, therefore, is to prepare the following information for your healthcare professional:

1. **Gather and send all prior medical records – such as office visit notes, blood lab reports, cultures, past surgeries, and CT scans – well in advance of your appointment.** This is in addition to filling out any pre-appointment forms and having your health insurance card on hand, and it can be particularly important when going to a new doctor for the first time. If you are an established patient and have signed a release allowing your providers to share information, your doctors will often share records electronically ahead of your appointment.

I believe the objective medical data is more important than the office visit notes, per se, because this allows the next healthcare provider to make their own independent interpretation, which he or she would do anyway. One physician I went to once suggested he only wanted to see CT scans and not the reports that accompany them. However, the office visit notes can and do offer useful context and are often requested.

Depending on the complexity of your condition and how many doctors you have seen, this could take *weeks* to gather, even though electronic sharing of information has made this process much faster and easier. You may need to make a few calls with your providers on the best way to have them send information, whether by fax, electronically, or by air mail. You want your doctor to have all the relevant information ahead of time so you can enjoy the most efficient use of your appointment time. That said, keep in mind that some doctors will review this information while others will not.

Furthermore, it has been my experience that sending your healthcare professional a brief personal note with a few key points of information may not effectively convey your concerns, as medical professionals are very busy and generally seem more attuned to our medical charts, official records, and prior healthcare provider notes. Consequently, while some doctors may in fact read your notes, many others will not. It has happened more than a few times that I sent a short, but what I thought was real important summary of my key issues, only to learn that the doctor did not read the note. So I had to re-explain the key issues at the appointment.

2. **Write down your list of *all* current medications and supplements, including the exact dosages and how often you take them.** *This is for your safety.* Taking medications from the same class, taking the wrong dose of a medication, or taking

two medications that adversely interact with each other are examples of potential problems, to name just a few. In fact, in the United States, adverse drug events (ADEs) lead to nearly 3.5 million physician office visits, 1 million emergency room visits, and 125,000 hospitalizations each year.[1]

The good news is that many of these ADEs are completely preventable, particularly if you simply share your current medications and supplements, including exact dosages, with your healthcare professionals. Furthermore, your doctor knows that you, like the majority of their patients, take a supplement and you do not want it to interact with your medications. So tell them everything. Also tell them any relevant alternative therapies you have tried.

After all, it is important for your healthcare professional to know exactly what you have tried – which is likely a lot. Doctors like to know that first-line treatments such as rest, heat, ice, and acetaminophen for chronic pain, for instance, have been tried prior to considering prescription pain medication. By telling your doctor what you have tried, the doctor will not only be clued in to what you have already done, but might be more inclined to recommend a more effective alternative, including an opioid medication, if needed.

As an aside, as a chronically ill patient you likely take multiple medications and require care from different providers. As a result, you will likely find yourself spending more than your fair share of time corresponding with pharmacists, your provider's offices, your insurance company, and even the blood lab to ensure that proper transmission of information has occurred. Expect to play a role in facilitating communication between multiple parties. All too often, prescription errors, communication breakdowns between doctor's offices, between the doctor's office and the pharmacy, between the doctor's office and the insurance company, between the insurance company and the pharmacy, and auto-generated messages from any of the above, will require your full attention and vigilance.

Rest assured that most of the time these errors will get corrected with patience, kindness, time and explanation – and a few phone calls. Despite the obstacles, the end result of a correctly prescribed medication and understanding provider is well worth it for your health.

Sample Medication Card

Medication/ Supplement Dose Frequency	Reason for taking	Effective	Side Effects	Prescriber
Zyrtec 10 mg 1x/daily	Allergies	Yes Strong	Drowsy	Dr. Smith
Amoxicillin 500 mg 2x/daily	Bacterial Infection	Yes Strong	Oral thrush; diarrhea	Dr. Urtz
Vitamin D3 2,000 IU 1x/daily	Vitamin D Deficiency	Yes Moderate	None	Dr. Ossont
Magnesium Citrate 200 mg 2x/daily	Stress Relief	Yes Strong	Laxative	Dr. Jaquay

3. **Consider inviting a second set of ears to your appointment, such as a family member or friend.** Research has shown that we patients only remember about *half* of the information and instructions provided to us at the doctor's appointment.[3] Stress

affects our memory and an office appointment can be stressful, particularly as we experience our healthcare ailment every second of every day and we want – and *need* – relief.

Let your family member or friend know how they can help you best in advance of the appointment. You may not want your friend to dominate the conversation – and to instead allow you the opportunity to explain your issues – but you also want him or her to speak or assert a point of view if something doesn't sound right or needs clarification.

Lastly, be sure to explain to your family member or friend your exact symptoms and how your symptoms affect your life, so they have a clear understanding of the problem.

4. **Prioritize your list of important questions.** Keep this list brief. You want to stay laser-focused on what is most important to you, and you should present your most important questions near the start of an appointment. Doing this ensures that your doctor addresses your most pressing questions. Assume each question you ask will take five minutes and your appointment will last 15 to 20 minutes.

5. **Identify your most pertinent symptom(s).** For each symptom, take note of the following:

- When your symptoms started. How long have you been dealing with your symptoms (e.g., 3 months)?
- The frequency of your symptoms. How often do you notice them per day?
- The duration of your symptoms. How long do they typically last?
- The severity of your symptoms. Is the severity low, moderate, or high?

◆ The precipitating factor(s). What happens before your symptoms begin?

◆ The alleviating factor(s). What makes your symptoms better?

You should identify all your symptoms, but if you can narrow down the symptoms as much as possible, then your doctor can stay more narrowly focused on your presenting concerns.

You should be very specific with your symptoms and identify them correctly, as a slightly different explanation of your symptoms can lead to a very different diagnosis. For example, I had a perplexing, intermittent, and uncontrolled symptom of temporomandibular joint (TMJ) pain for several years. I shared with multiple doctors that I had *ear pain* and this was consequently misdiagnosed as Eustachian tube dysfunction (ETD). Eventually, I shared that my pain was in *front of my ears* and I was *then* correctly diagnosed with TMJ. In collaboration with my healthcare providers, we tailored treatments to bring this symptom under control. It is now well-managed and has been for many years. Had I shared my symptom more specifically and accurately from the start, however, I would have been diagnosed and treated much earlier.

6. **Consider keeping (and then sharing) a diary of your symptoms.** This would not be a lengthy analysis of your symptoms, but simply note, for example, your pain, what triggers it, when it occurred, how long it occurred, its intensity on a 10-point scale, and what improves it. Another example is a sleep diary in which you record your sleep habits over a two-week period.

7. **Prepare an elevator speech.** Summarize your main presenting issues in half a minute or less. This speech should include the reason for referral, your main symptoms, and other pertinent life

circumstances that relate to your presenting concern such as a divorce, job loss, or a stressful life event. If your doctor already knows your needs, just focus on your health condition or symptom or medication.

For example, here is my elevator speech: "My nose and my lungs are compromised in their ability to clear mucus. The mucus is very thick. This contributes to more and longer lasting sinopulmonary infections and sleep-disordered breathing. As a result, I need to manually remove mucus through nasal washes, a nebulizer, and a vibrating vest. Additionally, I infuse daily with a therapy that provides my body with antibodies it cannot make on its own."

8. **Alternatively, if you already have a diagnosis, write down your chronic health condition, its associated signs and/or symptoms, and health goals.** For example, my immune deficiency disorder resulted in frequent sinus infections. My health goal was to reduce the rate of sinus infections from five per year to three or fewer per year.

9. **Determine the necessity for an appointment.** If you are dealing with a nagging symptom you and your doctor are familiar with, you could simply call (or email) your doctor's office and inquire whether a medication can be prescribed. I have done this to request medications for oral thrush, for example. If, on the other hand, your symptom has been lingering on and substantially limits your life activities – such as wrist pain that makes it too painful to type, tie your shoes, or lift objects – or your doctor simply wants to see you as it has been a while, then you should proceed to schedule an appointment.

Appointment Day Do's

1. **Arrive 15 to 20 minutes early.** This gives you time to fill out paperwork, use the bathroom, get basic vitals taken, and it may even allow for more time for the office visit. But remember: you might still wait for a while in the waiting room if your doctor is running behind because he or she is taking extra time with a different patient. That simply means he or she might also offer extra time for *you*.

2. **Make sure you can see and hear your doctor.** This may seem self-explanatory, but make sure to take your glasses with you to your appointment and/or your hearing aids, if you need them. Similarly, if your provider does not speak your native language, hire an interpreter to accompany you to your appointment.

3. **Describe your symptoms accurately.** Try to explain your symptoms exactly as they are, not minimizing or exaggerating them. Your doctors should know the exact symptoms, including side effects of medications or treatments, all of which can have a significant impact on your quality of life and the quality of treatment you receive. In fact, inaccurate reporting can lead to potential medication overdoses or interactions. It can be surprisingly harmful to lie – it is more harmful than you think.

   Keep in mind your word choice matters. For example, be very clear and specific about your symptoms. Is your pain dull, aching, or burning, or is it throbbing, piercing, and sharp? Your healthcare provider may interpret it differently depending on your exact wording.

   Furthermore, this is not a time to sugarcoat your experiences, as some might feel as though they are complaining or acting as a burden on the doctor, potentially taking away time from other patients who are supposedly in worse shape. Your health matters, too. You want your healthcare professional to know your exact symptoms so they can address and treat them.

4. **Describe your chronic illness experiences accurately.** You want your doctor to fully grasp the severity and impact of your chronic illness. Clearly describe how your illness impacts you in different aspects of your life. For instance, you could describe how your complex regional pain syndrome has impacted your work productivity, your relationships, and your ability to care for yourself on a daily basis.

5. *Always* **be respectful.** Stay calm, friendly, genuine, and open-minded. This factor, more than any other factor, will empower you in maintaining a positive rapport with your doctor.

According to Social Psychologists John French, PhD, and Bertram Raven, PhD, we can exert five types of power: *coercive power*, which uses fears and threats as incentives; *reward power*, which uses rewards as incentives; *legitimate power*, which derives from a job, position, or status; *expert power*, which derives from a high level of knowledge or specialized skill set; and *referent power*, which derives from reverence based on strong interpersonal skills. Guess which type of power is most potent? Referent power. With referent power, you can get anyone within your sphere of influence to do anything – within reason, of course. Former President George W. Bush excelled in referent power, and it was arguably a significant factor in delivering him the election in 2000.

6. **Listen attentively.** We generally do a better job of talking than listening. In fact, listening does not come naturally for most. We should strive to listen as best as we can.

7. **Speak up and ask questions for clarity, which improves your health literacy.** Clear communication is the key to understanding a diagnosis and following through on a treatment plan. In your attempt to ensure you understand medication directions, you might state, "So you want me to take two tablets each evening with food at the same time?" If you do not understand what your doctor said or need clarification, you must ask. I believe good healthcare professionals will honor and appreciate the person who humbly admits their lack of knowledge or understanding by trying to re-explain what they said. Health literacy, the ability to understand our health needs and healthcare plan, holds the key to successful implementation. We should aim to improve our health literacy.

8. **Honor your feelings.** This means knowing what you want and how you feel. Stated differently, trust your gut and/or your heart and go with it. You must respect yourself and your inner guidance so that you can get what you want and need. If your doctor seems to be avoiding or downplaying a topic or question you are attempting to ask, it is okay to be direct by stating, "This does not seem like an important matter to you. Why is that?" Then listen to what your doctor has to say.

9. **Ask "What else could this be?" when a diagnosis is made.** This allows your physician to avoid fixating on a diagnosis and instead consider alternate diagnoses.

10. **Be prepared for anything with respect to treatment options.** Some conditions may have a lot of treatment options while others have few evidence-based treatment options, or even none. The latter is more common for complex or rare conditions, and the latter can be quite disheartening. Try not to lose heart. Sometimes doing nothing can be the best option, or at least better than pursuing a risky treatment. Regardless,

continue to self-educate, seek additional opinions if desired, and keep an open mind to what can or cannot be done to manage your illness.

11. **Make small talk, but limit it.** Go ahead and make small talk and this will likely happen anyway, but remember that your doctor's time and *your* time is valuable. Bottom line: keep it focused, concise, and relevant.

12. **Assert your wants and needs.** For example, if you know you have tried every remedy in the book and your doctor is not coming up with new or alternative ideas, it's okay to state, "I would like to be considered for a higher dose of the opioid medication."

Appointment Day Don'ts

1. **Avoid discussing your concerns.** You need to address your concerns and you will regret it if you do not. Consider this: old age regret is typically centered around not what you have done in your life nor the mistakes you made, but what you did not do. What you avoided. The forgotten dreams. The wasted time. So speak up and address your concerns.

2. **Act disrespectful.** It is okay to disagree or point out a difference in opinion, as long as you do it in a respectful way. You could even take a mental note that this doctor might not be right for you. But if you are disrespectful, you may have just lost the most significant influence you may have over the doctor-patient relationship. This may also negatively influence your doctor's attitude toward you in the future when you need him or her.

3. **Complain about your previous physicians.** It may be tempting to be critical toward previous physicians you have been

to, particularly those who may have downplayed your concerns or you feel may have prevented you from accessing the care you need. You felt hurt and threatened by them. I understand. I have been there. But consider this: not only may your provider directly communicate with that doctor or put *their* interpretation of your complaint in your office visit notes, which will stay with *you* when you want to go to *another doctor*, but your doctor may also wonder what you will say about them next or even support another doctor – at your detriment. The doctor may also walk on eggshells with you or even try to avoid you. You never know if your comment could come back to haunt you in the future.

If you must relay what a previous provider had said as it holds direct relevance to your current symptoms, just stick to the facts and keep excessive emotions out of the discussion; rather, keep such emotions with trusted family, friends, or mental health professionals. Too much emotion might interfere with your doctor-patient relationship.

4. **Use your smartphone while your doctor is in the room.** Go ahead and use your phone while you are alone. You can even research information about what your doctor said. However, staying on the phone during the appointment distracts you and prevents you from listening and being fully engaged with your doctor, and it conveys disrespect to your doctor.

5. **Withhold relevant information.** Do not hide depression, alcohol use, or your incontinence. Your doctor cannot help you if he or she does not know what is happening. Withholding such information may prevent an accurate diagnosis or lead to a delay in necessary treatment.

6. **Demand that your physician complies with your requests.** Doctors do not need to submit to your requests, and asking for treatments, tests, referrals, and medications may prevent your

doctors from getting to the root of the problem. To make matters worse, your doctor may be even more resistant when you make perfectly reasonable requests.

7. **Act frustrated if shown to be wrong.** Physicians have undergone many years of extensive training to practice medicine – often up to eight years of college and then three or more years of residency. Yes, they make good money, but they have earned it through hard work and sacrifice. They have read countless texts, they have seen thousands of patients, and they have spent many sleepless nights endlessly learning their trade. This might be just so they can tie together unrelated symptoms and perhaps correctly diagnose *your* condition. So if your physician disagrees with you or points you to a different diagnosis, just relax, hold back, and keep an open mind. You may be wrong.

8. **Share subjective opinions, theories, or irrelevant information.** Like many with chronic illness, I am very analytical. I once shared the theory of how I believe I developed bronchiectasis over several years. However, while this information was very helpful in my understanding, it remained largely irrelevant to the current appointment, as my doctor appeared more focused on my current symptoms and what could be done about them. She did not want my full history and I would have saved both of us time by simply discussing my current symptoms.

In some cases, however, sharing succinct theories or opinions or extraneous detail could be beneficial if it is not time-consuming and does not confuse the doctor or distract him or her from focusing on what is most important, such as your most pressing symptoms.

After your Appointment

At the end of your appointment, many doctors will often provide a brief summary of the office visit and an "action plan" of what you need to do next, such as going for blood work or taking a new medication. Ask if you have questions. Otherwise – and this goes without saying – do what the plan says.

Other doctors may even automatically provide you with the office visit notes. If they do not and you are new to the doctor, have a question about the details of the appointment, want to ensure you did not miss anything, and/or want to ensure the doctor accurately understands your needs, you can also request a copy of the office visit notes. The office visit notes, after all, offer the most candid description of the appointment.

Occasionally upon reviewing office visit notes, I have noticed that a comment I made was quoted without proper context, the notes do not appear to grasp the big picture or severity of my symptoms, or they highlight a point of view I didn't realize the provider was trying to emphasize, such as a nurse practitioner recently recommending I promptly undergo an updated CT scan of my chest. These leave me feeling misunderstood. In any of these cases, it is okay to address them politely by email or a phone call, or preferably at the next appointment, depending on the seriousness of the error and the pertinence to our health.

When your Doctor is Wrong

Doctors are not God and they may – and will – misdiagnosis us at some point. The saying "to err is human, to forgive, divine" applies to how we should approach healthcare professionals. Healthcare professionals are people, too, and they will make diagnostic mistakes. We have to expect it. Their mistakes, however, can cost us time, money, and even our health.

One unfortunately common scenario is when our gut tells us there is something wrong, but the provider is minimizing the presenting concern or outright denying it. For example, a patient goes to a doctor complaining of a severe sore throat, but the doctor refuses to take a throat culture and outright denies the patient is suffering at all. The doctor might recommend to rest, to drink extra fluids, and to gargle with warm salt water. But untreated strep throat can lead to sinus infections, injury to the kidneys, and worse yet, Rheumatic fever, which can damage the heart, brain, and joints. So you must address your needs.

On the other hand, your doctor may seem dismissive, but is actually taking additional time to carefully investigate your presenting symptoms yet is having difficulty pinpointing the cause of your symptoms. While the perceived dismissiveness frustrates you right then, it is still an active effort to help.

As the patient, you should observe your relationship with your doctor and note whether your doctor genuinely seems to care and is listening to your concerns or acting dismissive, rude, or unhelpful on a regular basis. You might also note whether the dismissiveness or perceived callousness at an appointment are out of character for them. If out of character, cut them slack. If not, find another doctor.

Disagreement between specialists can present another obstacle when obtaining a clear diagnosis and treatment plan. This will likely happen. One doctor might diagnose one condition, but the next doctor might deny that same condition or may diagnose you with a different condition. This can lead to great patient confusion and anxiety. It is incumbent upon you, the patient, to seek care that gets to the root of your health condition.

While many patients prefer doctors to make the decisions on their healthcare, we patients hold ultimate responsibility for our health and should act as critical participants on our healthcare team. So do your research and stay with the provider whom you trust, and whose explanations make the most sense to you and are most consistent with your experience.

Get a Second Opinion

When your concerns are minimized, denied, or not adequately addressed, the first course of action should be to respectfully address your concerns directly with your doctor. But the buck should not stop there. Yet when faced with a major medical decision, about 70% of Americans do not feel compelled to seek a second opinion.[4] If your doctor is not listening to your concerns and your gut tells you the doctor-patient relationship is going downhill, I strongly recommend getting a second (or even third or more) opinion until your problem is correctly diagnosed. Your persistence in getting to the root of the matter is well worth it. And ironically, your first doctor will often welcome the second opinion. If your first doctor does not and acts highly defensive and/or dismissive, then you *know* you made the right decision in getting a second opinion.

Getting that second opinion is often warranted for patients with complex health needs. Trust your gut in deciding whether to trust your first doctor's opinion or to seek a second one. I believe when you are seeking a second opinion you should try to access the physician with the most reputable medical care you can find. Research online reviews on the providers, but take negative reviews with a grain of salt unless if they are overwhelmingly negative. Ask others for their experiences. Then seek care from your desired healthcare professional, if you can. This might mean, for example, a chronic pain sufferer seeking the most knowledgeable pain specialist in the area, or even going out of the area to seek knowledgeable medical care.

I live in Upstate New York, but was fortunate to have received outstanding medical care from a well-known immunologist who was a 4-hour drive for me. Despite some diagnostic confusion from my local providers, that immunologist promptly diagnosed me with a primary immune deficiency disorder and, more recently, his radiologist diagnosed me with bronchiectasis. These accurate diagnoses have empowered me to not only be understood accurately by all current and future doctors, but have also enabled me to access treatments that would have otherwise been unavailable. I have never for a moment regretted traveling to him for many years.

Thanks to my former immunologist's early and correct diagnosis, now that he is semi-retired, my care has been smoothly transitioned to another outstanding immunologist who is a 1 ½ hour drive.

I have also received exceptional surgical care from a renowned ear, nose, and throat (ENT) specialist who was an 8 ½ hour drive. That ENT specialist made modifications to my existing surgical implants for ENS, which has improved my nasal breathing. In fact, my nasal breathing has improved to the point that I am no longer seeking surgical care for ENS. Again, traveling for his medical care was well worth it.

The good news is with the increasing use of telehealth – video or phone visits – you may be able to access certain routine healthcare appointments from home. I personally have enjoyed some telehealth visits with my immunologist, which has cut down my travel time and expenses.

I would like to add an additional consideration when seeking medical care: many physicians are *sub-specialists within the specialties*. For example, a majority of allergists primarily devote most of their practice to treating allergies and asthma, but treat few patients with an immune deficiency disorder; conversely, my immunologist treats more than 100 patients with immune deficiencies. Likewise, among ENTs, some may have extra emphasis and training in managing ear conditions and putting in cochlear implants, others may have a focus on endoscopic sinus surgery, while still others may emphasize plastic surgery. So, assuming you have received an official diagnosis, you need to select the particular specialist carefully so he or she addresses your specific needs.

Does not Alternative Medicine Offer Quality Healthcare?

Absolutely! However, I believe that while alternative medicine does indeed offer quality healthcare, often with more of a personal touch than conventional medical care, it remains supplemental in nature. In many cases, it cannot replace medical care but rather should add to it, as the data is just not well-established in controlled human studies. I personally benefit from the best of both worlds.

The main advantage to conventional medical care is its research base. This is a big advantage. The conventional medical world has a strong scientific foundation of double-blind, placebo-controlled research studies. While the side effects of medicines and surgeries are generally greater with conventional medicine than the side effects of alternative medicine treatments, the benefits are well-studied and, therefore, more guaranteed; there is still plenty of failure in conventional medical treatments, of course.

Many people who battle chronic illnesses turn to natural medicine when they feel conventional medicine has failed them. Some alternative medicine proponents argue that conventional medicine is sick care, as the medicine treats the symptoms but does not address the root of the problem, thereby not allowing your body to heal itself over time. They further assert that conventional medicine is much better at treating acute or emergency illnesses rather than chronic illnesses. The conventionally trained specialist will look only at a very specific body part in a reductionist manner, they will note, not recognizing the holistic approach – that our body functions as a system of interdependent organs that all interact with and relate to each other. While all this makes sense in theory, I personally prefer to take advantage of the holistic benefits from alternative medicine while also enjoying the standardized benefits of conventional medicine.

My personal experiences with alternative medicine have been very positive, for the most part. I have gained benefit through acupuncture, craniosacral therapy, herbal remedies, and various supplements, for example. I have even had all my mercury amalgam fillings replaced with resin composites and porcelain onlays. I have explored nutritional therapy with gusto.

An Excellent Alternative Option: Chiropractic Care

Chiropractic care offers a valuable alternative medicine option, and insurance often covers this drug-free, surgery-free option. A typical chiropractic session involves lying face down on a padded chiropractic table, and the chiropractor applies a controlled, sudden force to a spinal joint which pushes it beyond its normal range of motion. Then the patient flips over on their back and the chiropractor applies additional adjustments. Despite the popping or cracking sounds you hear during the adjustment, it does not hurt. More importantly, the treatment is well worth it.

Research shows that spinal manipulation, while it can help many conditions, is particularly effective for low back and neck pain, as well as for headaches.[5] Recent research by chiropractor and neurophysiologist, Heidi Haavik, PhD, has been particularly instrumental in providing evidence of chiropractic care's effects on the central nervous system.[6]

I have been going to a wonderful chiropractor for the past 12 years, and I have found his adjustments to be very effective, for example, at alleviating lower back pain.

Three Considerations on Alternative Medicine

While I am a strong proponent of alternative medicine and have benefited much from it over the years, I believe it is wise for the chronically ill to consider the following:

1. **Do not seek alternative medicine exclusively and completely avoid conventional medical care.** In so doing, you may be avoiding necessary treatments that can help you. I will share that I have lost *years* by not pursuing proper medical help as I extensively exhausted only numerous natural remedies first. Do not make the same mistake as me. Some of the medicines I now take for managing my bronchiectasis have been tremendously helpful, such as Symbicort®.

2. **Conventional medical professionals sometimes recommend or offer natural remedies.** For example, sleep physicians routinely prescribe continuous positive airway pressure (CPAP) machine, which is nothing more than air and/or water that helps open up your airway during your sleep. An ear, nose and throat doctor recommends daily nasal saline washes. A pulmonologist recommends nebulized saline and/or a high frequency chest wall oscillation (HFCWO) vest to help clear your lower airways. A cardiologist recommends extensive movement throughout the day. An orthopedic surgeon puts on a cast to immobilize a broken bone.

3. **Do not overspend on alternative medicine if you are not seeing results.** Because the government does not subsidize many types of alternative medicine, it is often not covered by insurance. Consequently, you can easily overspend on various supplements when you are trying to treat your health, particularly if you have a challenging or complex health condition. Too many supplements are overhyped and underdeliver. They might be researched extensively through in

vitro studies (outside of living organisms) or through animal studies, but in general, they just are not well-researched on humans to treat specific conditions. Plus, supplements cannot take the place of a healthy diet, as the effects of a healthy diet are almost always stronger than supplements.

Personally, I take a small number of supplements that seem to have a solid research base such as vitamin D, magnesium, probiotics, fish oil, and N-Acetylcysteine. These supplements work slowly and over time. But I have also tried many supplements that appeared to do little for me. So be wise with your money and try not to overspend on natural medicine. And definitely share what you are taking with your doctor to prevent interactions with any conventional medicines you may be taking, or because you may need to go off them for a period of time before a surgery.

A conventionally trained physician may dismiss supplements and natural remedies as unproven therapies with no effectiveness. An alternative health care provider may suggest that conventional medicine poses too many risks. I believe the truth is somewhere in between, and I am thankful to enjoy the best of both worlds.

YOU are in the Driver's Seat

We take the greatest level of responsibility for our health of anyone. While we depend on others for help and support, only we can live our life and we therefore carry the greatest level of responsibility for its quality. This is especially true for those of us with invisible chronic illnesses.

In reference to the braggadocio shown in the War of 1812, Walt Kelly coined the phrase, "We have met the enemy and he is us." On the flip side, while the enemy might be us, we must also recognize that we can be our own best health advocates, as we are placed in the driver's seat of our lives.

Among other things, we can:

- ◆ Take ownership of our health conditions by accepting our chronic illness, by managing it effectively, and by using key psychological strategies to facilitate our mental and physical health.

- ◆ Embrace positive psychology while understanding its limitations. Staying positive can go a long way, and there is an abundance of research showing its efficacy, although we should also acknowledge it will not cure our invisible chronic illness.

- ◆ Manage stress through mindfulness, breathing techniques, exercise, and/or nature-based activities.

- ◆ Seek social support, as we invisible chronic illness sufferers need each other and we are "all in this together."

- ◆ Inform family, friends, and our healthcare professionals about our chronic illness to improve our relationships with them, and facilitate their awareness and acceptance of our condition.

- ◆ Empower our providers to make correct diagnoses and treatments through our own research and good communication skills.

We take ultimate responsibility for our lives. While we cannot change the past, we can take charge of our present and the future. In acting on the above, I believe we have the power to take our health to a whole new level. Despite how serious or challenging our chronic illness can be, we do not need to be defined or excessively limited by it.

Rather, we can use our chronic illness to gain a unique appreciation and perspective on life that others may take for granted, find new opportunities through our illness, and embrace the silver linings in even the darkest hours. By so doing, our health may improve and we may be able to live life to the fullest. Yes, we can live more abundantly.

Chapter 10

Eat a Healthy Diet

Y ou likely have heard the saying "You cannot out exercise a bad diet," which implies that no amount of exercise will undo the effects of eating unhealthy. You might also be aware of the "80 percent nutrition, 20 percent fitness rule," which means that your nutrition plays a much larger role than exercise for your health, although both remain important. Diet is clearly very important for your health.

Eating a healthy diet is a critical part of managing a chronic illness, as eating the wrong foods can cause flare-ups, while eating healthy foods can maintain your health. As Hippocrates, the founder of Western medicine said, "Let food be thy medicine, and medicine be thy food."

An enormous amount of information has been researched about food and its relation to health. Between fad diets, constantly changing nutritional recommendations, and a vast amount of research, it can be daunting for a chronically ill patient to figure out the ideal diet. Most with chronic illness have tried numerous diet plans and/or food modifications in attempt to improve their symptoms. For example, I have personally attempted a Paleolithic diet (meat and vegetable diet), an anti-candida diet (anti-yeast diet), as well as the ALCAT food rotation diet based on immunoglobulin G (IgG) food sensitivities, all in an attempt to improve my health.

Yet I believe the answer to nurturing our health and chronic illness through diet is surprisingly simple. *New York Times* bestselling author Michael Pollan summed it up in seven words: "Eat foods. Not too much. Mostly plants."

Ten Basic Tips for Eating Healthy with a Chronic Illness

In the same way, dietary considerations for those with chronic illness can be broken down into ten practical tips. The following list is not exhaustive or comprehensive, but boils down to some research-based considerations:

1. **Eat whole foods.** As Michael Pollan recommends, eat foods with five or fewer ingredients. The more ingredients a food has, the more processed it is.

2. **Eat five to nine servings of fruits and vegetables per day.** This is the United States Department of Agriculture (USDA) recommendation. I would add eat more vegetables than fruits because of the high sugar content in fruits.

3. **Eat in moderation.** Do not eat more than your digestive tract can handle. The Japanese term hara hachi bu means we should eat until about 80% full. We cannot know with certainty how full we are because our brains remain about 10 to 20 minutes behind our stomachs. So if you suspect you are 80% full, you may be 100% full.

4. **Drink water.** Water is a universal solvent, as it can break down more substances than any other liquid, and is often considered the healthiest beverage. I installed a reverse osmosis system in our house to reduce the contaminants in our water, so my family and I can drink purified water on a daily basis. Conversely, limit or eliminate high sugar drinks such as processed fruit juices and soda.

5. **Consume primarily complex carbohydrates.** Limit refined carbohydrates such as white sugar, high fructose corn syrup, and brown sugar. Examples of foods with complex carbohydrates

include rice, oatmeal, and potatoes. Additionally, on the topic of carbohydrates, research shows low carbohydrate diets can help in the management of chronic illnesses such as Type 2 diabetes. Of course, if you require a gluten-free diet or have Crohn's disease, for instance, you will need to avoid certain grains.

6. **Limit your meat intake, especially red meats.** Researchers have indicated a high intake of red and processed meats increase your risk for heart disease, cancer, diabetes, and an early death. I believe it is indeed fine to eat meat in general, as meat can provide vitamins and minerals you cannot get through plants, but avoid eating too much meat, particularly red meat.

Additionally, too much protein can be harmful for you, particularly on your kidneys.[1]

7. **Eat foods with resistant starch.** Most carbohydrates are starches, but not all starches get digested. Hence the term resistant starch. Rather, resistant starch acts like soluble fiber and feeds the friendly bacteria in your gut. Examples of resistant starch include oatmeal, unripened (green) bananas, and white and kidney beans.

8. **Eat fermented vegetables.** Fermented foods contain rich sources of good bacteria, often a much higher quantity than you can obtain through probiotic capsules, which have various health benefits including improved digestion and immunity. I personally enjoy eating a few ounces of kimchi on a daily basis. Other examples of fermented foods include yogurt, kefir, kombucha, and miso.

9. **Limit your sweets.** Limit your intake of those foods found to be universally unhealthy such as certain desserts, cake, or candy.

10. **Eat at least 80% healthy foods.** Go ahead and indulge on an occasional sweet, as it is easier to stick with a healthy diet that includes at least some cheating.

The Mediterranean Diet

The Mediterranean diet traces its origins from coastal Italy, Crete, and Greece in the 1960s where chronic disease was among the lowest in the world and adult life expectancy was among the highest. Developed in the 1960s to reduce the rate of heart disease, the Mediterranean diet has 50 years of research under its belt, is endorsed by the American Heart Association, and the US News and World Report has consistently ranked it as the #1 best overall diet.

Many studies have linked this diet to a lower risk of heart disease, stroke, obesity, and diabetes. Additionally, due to the high omega-3 fatty acid intake found in fish, research shows this diet not only contributes to lower rates of depression, but also reduces swelling and pain in rheumatoid arthritis.[2-4]

I personally strive to incorporate this diet, which I find delicious, flexible, diversified, budget-friendly, and thus easy to follow. The Mediterranean diet is a food eating plan without portion restrictions or a limit on calories.

The Mediterranean diet includes the following foods on a *daily basis*:

- Fresh fruits and vegetables.
- Olive oil. This is used in place of butter.
- Whole grains. Examples are brown rice, quinoa, and whole wheat bread.
- Nuts and seeds. Examples are almonds, walnuts, pistachios, pumpkin seeds, and flaxseeds.
- Legumes and beans.

♦ Herbs and spices.

The following foods are recommended a *few times per week*:

♦ Fish and chicken.
♦ Dairy, such as eggs, cheese, and yogurt.
♦ Wine.

Conversely, the following foods are recommended to be eaten *sparingly*:

♦ Sweets.
♦ Red meat.

An Adrenal Gland-Friendly Diet

Chronic illness sufferers often deal with chronic physical stress. As a result, it is possible they suffer from adrenal fatigue (which is not to be confused with Addison's disease, an adrenal insufficiency condition that is more severe and more widely accepted among the medical community). The adrenal glands are small glands that sit on top of the kidneys and secrete hormones, such as cortisol. Adrenal fatigue refers to the fact that the adrenal glands – when stressed – become overworked and may fail to produce enough hormones.

Although adrenal fatigue is not an accepted medical diagnosis, I believe that, given the physical and psychological stress associated with chronic illness, dietary strategies that benefit our adrenal glands merit consideration.

Six adrenal gland-friendly dietary considerations are:

1. Combine a fat, protein, and an unrefined complex carbohydrate food at each meal.

2. Eat breakfast before 10:00 A.M.

3. People with adrenal fatigue are often thirsty. Yet they can drink a lot of water, but still not get the hydration they need. This is because the hormone aldosterone – which is tasked with regulating water levels and the concentration of minerals in our bodies – is reduced. Consequently, sufferers of adrenal fatigue may excrete important minerals from their body.

One way to remediate this is to add ¼ to ½ teaspoon of sea salt – the most natural type of salt which contains over 80 minerals – to drinks of water. Because adrenal fatigue sufferers have low blood pressure, usually adding salt is not going to increase it significantly, although you can purchase a sphygmomanometer (blood pressure cuff) if you are concerned.

4. Eat low glycemic index fruit such as apples, pears, and cherries.

5. Eat vegetables, half of them raw, and particularly the brightly colored ones. Examples are Brussels sprouts, carrots, peppers, sweet potatoes, and broccoli.

6. Avoid coffee and chocolate. Although black coffee and dark chocolate do have health benefits and are high in antioxidants – chemicals that stop or limit free radical damage – both adversely affect the adrenal glands.

For additional recommendations on addressing adrenal fatigue, an excellent resource is *Adrenal Fatigue: The 21st Century Stress Syndrome*, which was written in 2001 but is just as applicable today.

Chapter 11

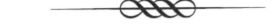

Embrace Your New Normal

U nderstanding or learning about much of the information in *Finding Joy* is easy, and hopefully enjoyable. You easily understand acceptance, self-compassion, positive reappraisal, positive self-talk, pacing, social support, and the various positive psychology concepts and stress management techniques, for example.

Yet changing your ways by putting them into practice over the long haul remains the challenge. Do not despair. Taking on a new behavior over a long period of time can be challenging due to our tendencies toward maintaining the status quo. However, change is within your reach and the trick lies in creating a new habit.

Here is how you create that new habit. Once you have done an activity over and over, such as at your work place or volunteer work duties, or your making of a meal or driving to work, it becomes easier and much more automatic with practice. Creating this new habit or habits can take days, weeks, or months to become automatic. But eventually, you do these behaviors again and again in an autopilot mode. It becomes the most challenging to maintain these new habits between the 3rd and 7th week, so it is important to do whatever you can to keep going and stay motivated during this time period. By staying motivated and continually putting that behavior into practice past this time period, you will have successfully create a new habit.

It is best to focus your energy on one, two, or even three principles or strategies in this book that you know you need to improve in your life. If you try to put them all into practice immediately, you will set yourself up for failure and become the "jack of all trades, master of none." We succeed where we focus.

For instance, upon finishing the writing of *Finding Joy*, I decided I would like to laugh more in my life by watching humorous shows or reading the comics, as well as apply the breathing techniques to improve my lower respiratory breathing. So my focus will remain on these two strategies, which I will schedule for 15 minutes each day for at least the next two months.

So go ahead and do the same by selecting a strategy or two or three, pencil in when and how much time you will implement it per day, and take action by creating a new habit. You can do it.

For further information on creating new positive habits, read *Atomic Habits: An Easy & Proven Way to Build Good Habits & Break Bad Ones.* In this outstanding guidebook, *#1 New York Times* bestselling author James Clear equips you to make those tiny changes to your habits, which lead to remarkable results over the long-term.

In closing, as a result of your invisible chronic illness, your life has changed with newfound limitations and challenges, but also with new and unique opportunities for personal, physical, and spiritual growth. By changing your thinking, feelings, and behaviors through realistic expectations, improved moods, and newfound habits, you can enjoy the high quality of life you deserve. The mind is a terrible thing to waste but, if used correctly, will take you places.

Your life does not boil down to a diagnosis nor does this diagnosis define you; rather, you effectively manage this aspect of your life. But your invisible chronic illness does represent your new normal with its flare-ups and remissions. It is up to you to adapt to and embrace this new normal as best you can.

Knowing how hard and how much you have already accomplished just by merely enduring an invisible chronic illness, I believe you will no doubt rise to this challenge. Considering your impressive persistence, determination, and victories, you have already achieved warrior status in my mind. You are tough. You are a fighter. And there is always a silver lining in every battle you fight.

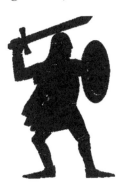

Bibliography

Introduction References

1. US and World Population Clock. Retrieved January 16, 2021 from The United States Census Bureau Web site at: https://www.census.gov/popclock/.
2. Invisible Disabilities: List and General Information. Retrieved July 13, 2020, from the Disabled World Web site at: https://www.disabled-world.com/disability/types/invisible/.
3. Chronic Illness and Depression. Retrieved July 15, 2020, from the Cleveland Clinic Web site at: https://my.clevelandclinic.org/health/articles/9288-chronic-illness-and-depression.

Chapter 1 References

1. Hughes, L.S., Clark, J., Coclough, J.A., Dale, E., & McMillan, D. (2017). Acceptance and Commitment Therapy (ACT) for Chronic Pain: A Systematic Review and Meta-Analyses. *The Clinical journal of pain,* 33 (6): 552-568.
2. Sirois, F.M., Molnar, D.S., & Hirsch, J.K. (2015). Self-Compassion, Stress, and Coping in the Context of Chronic Illness. *Self and Identity,* 14 (3): 334-347.
3. Neff, K.D., Rude, S.S., & Kirkpatrick, K.L. (2007). 41 (2007) 908–916. An examination of self-compassion in relation to positive psychological functioning and personality traits. *Journal of Research in Personality,* 41: 908-916.
4. Self-compassion. Retrieved July 29, 2020 from the Self-compassion Web site at: https://self-compassion.org/the-three-elements-of-self-compassion-2/.
5. What is Positive Self-Talk. Retrieved July 31, 2020, from the Positivepsychology.com Web site at: https://positivepsychology.com/positive-self-talk/.
6. Hovenkamp-Hermelink, J.H.M., Jeronimus, B.F., Spinhoven, P., Penninx, B.W., Schoevers, R.A., & Riese, H. (2019). "Differential associations of

locus of control with anxiety, depression and life-events: A five-wave, nine-year study to test stability and change." *Journal of Affective Disorders*, 253, 26-34.

7. Goudsmit, E.M., Nijs, J., Jason, L.A., & Wallman, K.E. (2011). Disability Rehabilitation. 2012;34(13):1140-7.. Epub 2011 Dec 19. Pacing as a strategy to improve energy management in myalgic encephalomyelitis/chronic fatigue syndrome: a consensus document. *Disability Rehabilitation*, 34 (13): 1140-1147.

8. 'Leave it to Beaver' Star Hugh Beaumont was very much like on-screen family man, daughter says. Retrieved July 31, 2020, from the Fox News Web site at: https://www.foxnews.com/entertainment/leave-it-to-beaver-star-hugh-beaumont.

*Most of the research on treatments for chronic illness has been done on adult subjects, and therefore the results cannot be generalized to children.

Chapter 2 References

1. Park, N., Peterson, C., Szvarca, D., Vander Molen, R., Kim, E.S., & Collon, K. (2016). 2016 May-Jun; 10(3): 200–206. Positive Psychology and Physical Health Research and Applications. *American Journal of Lifestyle Medicine*, 10(3): 200-206.

2. Danner, D.D., Snowdon, D.A., & Friesen, V.W. Positive emotions in early life and longevity: findings from the nun study. *Journal of Personality and Social Psychology*, 80, 804-813.

3. Ghosh, A.. & Amrita, D. (2017). Positive Psychology Interventions for Chronic Physical Illnesses: A Systematic Review. *Psychological Studies*, 62 (3): 213-232.

4. Schiavon, C.C., Marchetti, E., Gurgel, L.G., Busnello, F.M., & Reppold, C.T. (2016). Optimism and Hope in Chronic Disease: A Systematic Review. *Frontiers in Psychology*, 7, 2016-2022.

5. Norem, J. K., & Burdzovic Andreas, J. (2006). Understanding journeys: Individual growth analysis as a tool for studying individual differences in change over time. In A. D. Ong & M. van Dulmen (Eds.), *Handbook of Methods in Positive Psychology* (pp. 1036-1058). London: Oxford University Press.

6. Norem, J.K. (2001). Defensive pessimism, optimism, and pessimism. In Chang, Edward (Ed). *Optimism & pessimism: Implication for theory, research, and*

practice (pp. 77–100). Washington DC: American Psychological Association.

7. Sone T, Nakaya N, & Ohmori K, et al. (2008). Sense of life worth living (ikigai) and mortality in Japan: Ohsaki study. *Psychosomatic Medicine*, 70, 709-715.

8. Chapman, B.P., Wijngaarden, E., Seplaki, C.L., Talbot, N., Duberstein, P., & Moynihan, J. (2011). Openness and conscientiousness predicts 32-week patterns of Interleukin-6 in older persons. *Brain, Behavior, and Immunity*, 25 (4): 667-673.

9. Qi, Q., Ailiyaer, Y., Liu, R., Zhang, Y., Li, C., Liu, M., Wang, X., Jing, L., & Li, Y. (2019). Effect of N-acetylcysteine on exacerbations of bronchiectasis (BENE): a randomized controlled trial. *Respiratory Research*, 20, 73.

10. Stilley CS, Sereika S, Muldoon MF, Ryan CM, Dunbar-Jacob, J (2004). Psychological and cognitive function: predictors of adherence with cholesterol lowering treatment. *Annals of Behavior Medicine*, 27(2): 117–24.

11. O'Cleirigh C, Ironson G, Weiss A, & Costa PT, Jr. (2007). Conscientiousness predicts disease progression (CD4 number and viral load) in people living with HIV. *Health Psychology*, 26(4): 473–80.

12. Steptoe, A., & Wardle, J. (2005). Positive affect and biological function in everyday life. *Neurobiology of Aging*, 26 (1): 108-112.

13. Marsland, A.L., Cohen, S., Rabin, B.S., & Manuck, S.B. (2006). Trait positive affect and antibody response to hepatitis B vaccination. *Brain, Behavior, and Immunity*, 20 (3), 261-269.

14. Papousek, I., Nauschnegg, K., Paechter, M., Lackner, H.K., Goswami, N., & Schulter, G. (2010). Trait and state positive affect and cardiovascular recovery from experimental academic stress. *Biological Psychology*, 83 (2): 108-115.

15. Finan, P.H., & Garland, E.L. (2015). The Role of Positive Affect in Pain and its Treatment. *Clinical Journal of Pain*, 31(2): 177–187.

16. Angner, E., Ghandhi, J., Williams Purvis, K., & Amante, D. (2012). Daily Functioning, Health Status, and Happiness in Older Adult. *Journal of Happiness Studies*. 14(5), 1563-1574.

17. Boggiss, A.L., Consedine, N.S., Brenton-Peters, J.M., Hofman, P.L., & Serlachius, A.S. (2020). A systematic review of gratitude interventions: Effects on physical health and health behaviors. *Journal of Psychosomatic Research*, 135, 110-165.

18. Sirois, F.M., & Wood, A.M. (2017). Gratitude uniquely predicts lower depression in chronic illness populations: A longitudinal study of inflammatory bowel disease and arthritis. *Health Psychology*, 36(2):122-132.

19. Bennett, M.P., & Lengacher, C. (2009). Human and Laughter May Influence Health IV. Humor and Immune Function. *Evidence- Based Complementary and Alternative Medicine*, 6(2): 159–164.

20. 5 Benefits of Healthy Relationships. Retrieved August 18, 2020 from the Northwestern Medicine Web site at: https://www.nm.org/healthbeat/healthy-tips/5-benefits-of-healthy-relationships.

21. Hatala, A.R., & Roger, K. (2017). Religion, Spirituality & Chronic Illness: A Scoping Review and Implications for Health Care Practitioners. *Journal of Religion & Spirituality in Social Work.*, 37, 24-44.

22. Forgiveness: Letting go of grudges and bitterness. Retrieved August 20, 2020 from the Mayo Clinic Web site at: https://www.mayoclinic.org/healthy-lifestyle/adult-health/in-depth/forgiveness/art-20047692.

23. Lawler, K.A., Younger, J.W., Piferi, R.L., Jobe, R.L., Edmondson, K.A., & Jones, W.H. (2005). The unique effects of forgiveness on health: an exploration of pathways. *Journal of Behavior Medicine,* 28 (2): 157-167.

24. How prayer and meditation can make you healthier. Retrieved August 20, 2020 from the Houston Chronicle Web site at: https://www.houstonchronicle.com/local/gray-matters/article/How-prayer-and-meditation-can-make-you-healthier-8329972.php.

25. Boelens, P.A., Reeves, R.R., & Replogle, (2010). A Randomized Trial of the Effect of Prayer on Depression and Anxiety. *The International Journal of Psychiatry in Medicine,* 39 (4): 377-392.

26. Post, S.G. (2005). Altruism, Happiness, and Health: It's Good to Be Good. *International Journal of Behavioral Medicine,* 12 (2): 66–77.

27. Hammond, C. (2004). Impacts of lifelong learning upon emotional resilience, psychological and mental health: fieldwork evidence. In *Oxford Review of Education,* 30 (4): 551-568.

Chapter 3 References:

1. Salleh, M.R. (2008). Life Event, Stress, and Illness. *Malaysian Journal of Medical Science*, 15(4): 9–18. Merkes, M. (2010). Mindfulness-based stress

reduction for people with chronic diseases. *Australian Journal of Primary Health*, 16(3):200-10.

2. How Mindfulness Can Ease Symptoms of Chronic Illness. Retrieved August 23, 2020 from the IG Living Web site at: http://www.igliving.com/magazine/articles/IGL_2017-06_AR_How-Mindfulness-Can-Ease-the-Symptoms-of-Chronic-Illness.pdf.

3. Ubolnuar, N., Tantisuwat, A., Thaveeratitham, P., Lertmaharit, S., Kruapanich, C., & Mathiyakom, W. (2019). Effects of Breathing Exercises in Patients with Chronic Obstructive Pulmonary Disease: Systematic Review and Meta-Analysis. *Annals of Rehabilitative Medicine,* 43(4): 509–523.

4. Zaccaro, A., Piarulli, A., Laurino, M., Garbella, E., Menicucci, D., Neri, B., & Gemignani, A. (2018). How Breath-Control Can Change Your Life: A Systematic Review on Psycho-Physiological Correlates of Slow Breathing. *Frontiers in Human Neuroscience*, 12, 353.

5. Santino, T.A., Chaves, G.S., Freitas, D.A., Fregonezi, G.A., Mendonça, K.M. (2020). Breathing exercises for adults with asthma. *The Cochrane Database of Systematic Reviews.*

6. Chu, L., Valencia, I.J., Garvert, D.W., & Montoya, J.G. (2018). Deconstructing post-exertional malaise in myalgic encephalomyelitis/chronic fatigue syndrome: A patient-centered, cross-sectional survey. *PLoS One*, 13, 6.

7. Eda, N. (2014). Yoga has Beneficial Effects on Patients with Chronic Diseases and Improves Immune Functions (2014). *Journal of Clinical Research & Bioethics*, 5 (5).

8. A Prescription for better health: go alfresco. Retrieved August 24, 2020 from the Harvard Health Newsletter, Harvard Medical School Web site at: https://www.health.harvard.edu/newsletter_article/a-prescription-for-better-health-go-alfresco.

9. Menigoz, W., & Sinatra, D. (2020). Integrative and lifestyle medicine strategies should include earthing (grounding): Review of research evidence and clinical observations. *Explore.* 16 (3): 152-160.

10. Soga, M., Gaston, K.J., & Yamaura, Y. (2017). Gardening is beneficial for health: A meta-analysis. *Preventive Medicine Reports*, 5, 92-99.

11. Pennebaker, J.W. (1997). Writing about emotional experiences as a therapeutic process. *Psychological Science*, 8(3):162-166.

12. Smyth, J.M. (1998). Written emotional expression: effect sizes, outcome types, and moderating variables. *Journal of Consulting and Clinical Psychology*, 66(1):174-184.

13. Baikie, K.A., & Wilhelm, K. (2005). Emotional and physical health benefits of expressive writing. *Advanced Psychiatric Treatments*, 11(5):338-346.

14. Van Emmerik, A.A., Reijntjes A, & Kamphuis JH (2013). Writing therapy for posttraumatic stress: a meta-analysis. *Psychotherapy and Psychosomatics*, 82(2):82-88.

15. Pennebaker JW. (2004). Writing to Heal: A Guided Journal for Recovering From Trauma & Emotional Upheaval. Oakland, CA: New Harbinger Publications.

16. Kennedy D.O., Veasey R., Watson A., Dodd F., Jones E., Maggini S., & Haskell C.F. (2010). Effects of high-dose B vitamin complex with vitamin C and minerals on subjective mood and performance in healthy males. *Psychopharmacology*, 211, 55–68.

17. 9 Herbs for anxiety. Retrieved August 30, 2020 from the Medical News Today Web site at: https://www.medicalnewstoday.com/articles/herbs-for-anxiety#chamomile.

18. Hoekstra, S. P., Bishop, N.C., Faulkner, S.H., Bailey, S.J., & Leicht, C.A. (2018). Acute and chronic effects of hot water immersion on inflammation and metabolism in sedentary, overweight adults, *Journal of Applied Physiology*, 125, 2008-2018.

Chapter 4 References

1. Lamberg L (1996). Treating depression in medical conditions may improve quality of life. *Journal of the American Medical Association*, 276: 857-858.

2. Panos P.T., Jackson J.W., Hasan O., & Panos A. (2014). Meta-analysis and systematic review assessing the efficacy of dialectical behavior therapy (DBT). *Research on Social Work Practice*, 24(2).

3. Cuijpers, P., Geraedts, A.S., van Oppen, P., Andersson, G., Markowitz, J.C., & van Straten, A. (2011). Interpersonal psychotherapy for depression: a meta-analysis. *American Journal of Psychiatry*, 168 (6), 581-592.

4. Shedler, J.K. (2010). The efficacy of psychodynamic psychotherapy. *American Psychologist*, Vol. 65. No.2.

5. Schema Therapy Institute. Retrieved February 17, 2021 from the Schema Therapy Institute Web site at: https://www.schematherapy.com.

6. Kindynis, S., Burlacu, S., Louville, P., & Limosin, F. (2013). Effect of schema-focused therapy on depression, anxiety, and maladaptive cognitive schemas in the elderly.

Chapter 5 References

1. Cockerham, W.C., Hamby, B.W., & Oates, G.R. (2017). The Social Determinants of Chronic Disease. *American Journal of Preventive Medicine*, 52 (1 Suppl 1): S5-S12.

2. Umberson D, & Montez J. (2010). Social relationships and health: a flashpoint for health policy. *Journal of Health and Social Behavior*, 51, S54–S66.

3. Taylor, S.E. (2007). Social support. In Friedman, H.S.; Silver, R.C. (eds.). *Foundations of health psychology*. New York: Oxford University Press, 145–171.

Chapter 6 Reference

1. 30 years after the ADA, access to voting for people with disabilities is still an issue. Jeanine Santucci. *USA TODAY*, July 26, 2020.

Chapter 7 References

1. Rees, J., O'Boyle, C., & MacDonagh, R. (2001). Quality of life: impact of chronic illness on the partner. *Journal of the Royal Society of Medicine*, 94, 11, 563-566.

2. Ng, R., Sutradhar, R., Yao, Z., Wodchis, W.P., & Rosella, L.C. (2020). Smoking, drinking, diet and physical activity—modifiable lifestyle risk factors and their associations with age to first chronic disease. *International Journal of Epidemiology*, Volume 49 (1): 113–130.

Chapter 9 References

1. US Department of Health and Human Services, Office of Disease Prevention and Health Promotion (ODPHP). Retrieved July 30, 2020, from the ODPHP Web site at: https://health.gov/our-work/health-care-quality/adverse-drug-events.

2. Average Time Doctors Spend with Patients: What's the Number for Your Physician Specialty? Debra Wood, RN. December 27, 2017. Staff Care.
3. McCarthy, D.M., Waite, K.R., Curtis, L.M., Engel, K.G., Baker, D.W., & Wolf, M.S. (2012). What Did the Doctor Say? Health Literacy and Recall of Medical Instructions. *Medical Care*, 50 (4): 277-282.
4. Five things you may not know about second opinions. Retrieved July 30, 2020 from the Harvard Health Publishing, Harvard Medical School Web site at: https://www.health.harvard.edu/press_releases/five-things-you-may-not-know-about-second-opinions.
5. LeFebvre, R., Peterson, D., & Haas, M. (2013). Evidence-Based Practice and Chiropractic Care. *Journal of Evidenced Based Complementary and Alternative Medicine*, 18 (1), 75-79.
6. Haavik H., Niazi I.K., Jochumsen M., Sherwin D., Flavel S., & Türker K.S. (2016). Impact of Spinal Manipulation on Cortical Drive to Upper and Lower Limb Muscles. *Brain Sciences*, 7(1): 2.

Chapter 10 References

1. When it comes to protein, how much is too much? Retrieved August 30, 2020, from the Harvard Health Publishing, Harvard Medical School Web site at: https://www.health.harvard.edu/nutrition/when-it-comes-to-protein-how-much-is-too-much.
2. Appleton KM, Sallis HM, Perry R, Ness AR, & Churchill R. (2015). Omega-3 fatty acids for depression in adults. *Cochrane Database Systematic Reviews*, 11, 1-120.
3. Proudman, J.M., & Cleland L. (2010). Fish oil and rheumatoid arthritis: past, present and future. *Proceedings of the Nutrition Society*, 69 (3), 316-323.
4. Goldberg RJ, & Katz J. (2007). A meta-analysis of the analgesic effects of omega-3 polyunsaturated fatty acid supplementation for inflammatory joint pain. *Pain*, 129, 210-223.

Acknowledgements

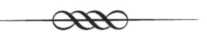

F irst and foremost, I would like to thank my Savior and Lord Jesus Christ for giving me strength, endurance, and compassion to write this book.

I would like to thank my beautiful wife, Colleen, who was supportive while I spent endless hours writing and thinking about this book. She also spent time reviewing the manuscript and offering constructive feedback, which greatly enhanced the finished product. She is a source of great support and inspiration to me, in good times and bad. I would also like to thank my daughters, Faith, Abigail, Charity, and Liberty, and my sons, Luke and Jacob, for their support as well.

I would like to thank my father who is a retired pharmacist after 50 years of service. His work ethic and dedication to profession is impressive and inspiring. Dad has accompanied me to many medical appointments over the years. I would also like to thank Mom who is wonderful and supportive. I have the best parents in the world.

I would like to thank Subinoy Das, MD, FACS, FARS. Dr. Das read this book, has been very encouraging, and wrote a terrific foreword. He is CEO and director of the US Institute for Advanced Sinus Care & Research.

I would like to thank Alla Bogdanova who offered me substantial and extensive feedback, insights, and numerous constructive suggestions throughout the book, which significantly enhanced the finished product. Her enthusiasm and passion for the message in this book, and dedication to those who suffer, is inspiring. Alla is co-founder and past president of the International Empty Nose Syndrome Association.

I would like to thank A. Phelps who offered me important feedback on both the technical and content aspects of this book. Her contributions, constructive suggestions, and support greatly enhanced the final product.

I would like to thank the team at word-2-kindle.com who performed high quality work of converting the print book into an eBook format. This team offered a rare and refreshing level of communication, responsiveness, professionalism, and attention to detail. Their expertise and flawless work resulted in a fantastic eBook.

I would like to thank Lance Buckley, a book cover designer at www.lancebuckley.com, along with his assistant Beth, who created an outstanding cover design. His expertise, dedication, and attention to detail greatly enhanced the finish product.

I would like to thank the following who read the book, and/or have offered feedback and support:

- ◆ Heather Lewis-Hoover, a cherished colleague and school counselor.
- ◆ James Nestor, *New York Times* bestselling author of *Breath: The New Science of a Lost Art.*
- ◆ Judith Rosinski, my outstanding physical therapist.
- ◆ Christopher Smith, MD, my superstar immunologist who excels in managing immune deficient patients. Dr. Smith is director of research at Smith Allergy & Asthma Specialists, and he is a nationally recognized author and researcher.
- ◆ Suzan Fenstermacher, RPA-C, my skilled and very caring and knowledgeable clinician at Smith Allergy & Asthma Specialists.
- ◆ Richard Loftus, MD, my compassionate and brilliant PCP who is perfect for managing complex chronic illness patients like me.

- Justin Zalatan, DDS, and Salina Suy, FAGD, DDS, my family's dedicated, outstanding dentists who go above and beyond in offering cutting-edge dental care.
- Mohammed Seedat, MD, my astute, witty, and supportive sleep doctor.
- Joseph LaBarbara, DC, my phenomenal and very effective chiropractor.

About the Author

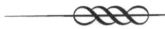

C hris Martin completed 7 years of college and is a nationally certified school psychologist (NCSP) in Upstate New York. He furthered his education in 2009 and earned a Certificate of Advanced Study (CAS) in school psychology.

In 2007, Chris published *Having Nasal Surgery? Don't You Become An Empty Nose Victim!* *Having Nasal Surgery?* won a 2008 Independent Publisher Book Award, Bronze Medalist, in Health/Medicine/Nutrition. In 2015, it was translated into Spanish by J.A. Guzmán under the title *¿Cirugía nasal? ¡No caiga en las garras del síndrome de la nariz vacía!*

Despite living with multiple invisible chronic illnesses for the past 25 years and knowing how tough they can be, Chris still considers himself tremendously blessed because he is married to his amazing wife Colleen, and has four daughters and two sons (from left to right) (front): Charity & Liberty; (back): Luke, Abigail, Faith, & Jacob.

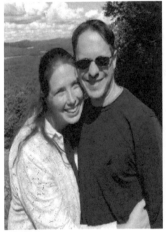
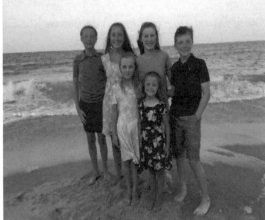

Make My Day

If you enjoyed this book, the best way you can thank me is to take just a few moments to write a review on Amazon.com. You could mention how this book could help potential readers, how this book helped you, and who specifically this book could benefit.

By leaving a review on Amazon, the world's largest bookstore, you can make a tremendous difference in helping potential readers discover *Finding Joy*. Doing so would literally make my day and I would feel extremely grateful. Thank you!

Lastly, to get the most out of *Finding Joy*, consider using the *Workbook for Christopher Martin's Finding Joy with an Invisible Chronic Illness* at Amazon.com. This could be useful for personal application or in a support group or book club.

Other Books by Christopher Martin

Having Nasal Surgery? Don't You Become An Empty Nose Victim!

¿Cirugía nasal? ¡No caiga en las garras del síndrome de la nariz vacía! (Spanish Translation)

Made in United States
Troutdale, OR
02/21/2024

17849401R10116